T0074196

The Achilles Tendon

Hajo Thermann • Christoph Becher
Michael R. Carmont • Jón Karlsson
Nicola Maffulli • James Calder
C. Niek van Dijk
Editors

The Achilles Tendon

An Atlas of Surgical Procedures

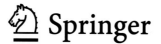

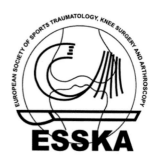

Editors
Hajo Thermann
Center for Hip, Knee and Foot Surgery
ATOS Clinic Centre
Heidelberg
Germany

Christoph Becher
Center for Hip, Knee and Foot Surgery
ATOS Clinic Centre
Heidelberg
Germany

Michael R. Carmont
Princess Royal Hospital
Telford
Shropshire
UK

Jón Karlsson
Sahlgrenska Academy
University of Gothenburg
Mölndal
Sweden

Nicola Maffulli
Department of Medicine and Surgery
University of Salerno
Fisciano
Salerno
Italy

James Calder
Chelsea and Westminster Hospital
London
UK

C. Niek van Dijk
Dept of Orthopaedic Surgery
Academic Medical Centre
Amsterdam Zuidoost
The Netherlands

ISBN 978-3-662-54073-2   ISBN 978-3-662-54074-9   (eBook)
DOI 10.1007/978-3-662-54074-9

Library of Congress Control Number: 2017936675

Printed on acid-free paper

This Springer imprint is published by Springer Nature
The registered company is Springer-Verlag GmbH Germany
The registered company address is: Heidelberger Platz 3, 14197 Berlin, Germany

Preface

The publication of a detailed operating atlas for Achilles tendon surgery is logically consistent with the three previously published books, which reflected the pathologies, treatment concepts and results based on the latest standard.

The special feature of this atlas is being the contribution of globally renowned Achilles tendon surgeons, who present their specific approach to various pathologies and their personal techniques.

So it is as if we were looking over the shoulder of the "masters".

The format of the book is selected in such a way that the most important steps in a surgical procedure and its technical execution are standardised and easily reproducible in each chapter. The authors are mainly concerned with setting, the indications as well as demonstration of technical tricks within the scope of the operation, which – in our opinion – were not emphasised in the literature.

Our major concern is the reflection of the "Pearls and Pitfalls" which raises the attention of the surgeon to these particular highlights in order to improve the results and to avoid encountering the mistakes that we all have behind us.

The compilation of the international authors can only go beyond the editors in such an atmosphere in order to achieve an absolutely international "top-ranking spectrum" for this book.

We also wanted to underline the uniqueness of this book through the artistic presentation. The pictures by Mr. Jörg Kühn in our view are extraordinary and represent the details in high quality. The cooperation between the authors and the artist has been carried out purposefully in order to illustrate the carried-out operations thoroughly. The editors would like to thank all the authors involved for the participation and the expertise and the transfer of knowledge.

Special thanks go to Dr. Christoph Becher, PhD, who has been the "working horse" for organisation, communication and review. Special thanks also go to Mike Carmont, who has improved the linguistic style for the non-native speakers once again with excellent Oxford English.

All in all, the editors are happy that an operative standard work has been created, which will hopefully serve all Achilles tendon surgeons as a "vade mecum" to improve their surgical skills.

In contrast to previous other books, this book has already included the minimally invasive and the endoscopic Achilles tendon surgery, so that it can already be a "door opener" for every surgeon who will turn to these techniques, which will play an outstanding role in the future.

Heidelberg, Germany   Hajo Thermann
                                                      Christoph Becher
Telford, Shropshire, UK   Michael R. Carmont
Molndal, Sweden   Jón Karlsson
Fisciano, Salerno, Italy   Nicola Maffulli
London, UK   James Calder
Amsterdam Zuidoost, The Netherlands   C. Niek van Dijk

Contents

Part I   Acute Achilles Tendon Ruptures: Suture Techniques

1   **Open Standard Technique**   3
Jon Karlsson, Nicklas Olsson, Michael R. Carmont,
and Katarina Nilsson-Helander

2   **Percutaneous Suturing with a Double-Knot Technique**   7
Hajo Thermann and Christoph Becher

3   **Three-Bundle Technique**   15
Gwendolyn Vuurberg and C. Niek van Dijk

4   **Lace Technique Modified by Segesser and Weisskopf**   21
Lukas Weisskopf and Anja Hirschmüller

5   **Achillon® Achilles Tendon Suture System**   27
Andrew J. Roche and James D. F. Calder

6   **Repair of Distal Achilles Tendon Rupture
and Reattachment**   31
Michael R. Carmont, Gordon Mackay, and Bill Ribbans

Part II   Mid Portion Tendinopathy

7   **Open Debridement of Mid-Portion Achilles Tendinopathy** . . .   39
Katarina Nilsson-Helander, Nicklas Olsson,
Olof Westin, Michael R. Carmont, and Jon Karlsson

8   **Endoscopic Debridement**   45
Hajo Thermann and Christoph Becher

Part III   Insertional Tendinopathy

9   **Open Technique**   53
Lukas Weisskopf, Patric Scheidegger, Th. Hesse, H. Ott,
and A. Hirschmüller

10   **Endoscopic Technique for Noncalcified Tendinopathy**   61
K. T. M. Opdam, J. I. Wiegerinck, and C. Niek van Dijk

11   Open Technique for Calcified Insertional
     Achilles Tendinopathy   69
     Paul G. Talusan and Lew C. Schon

Part IV   Delayed Reconstruction of Achilles Tendon Rupture

12   Open Reconstruction with Gastrocnemius
     V-Y Advancement....................................   75
     Andrew R. Hsu, Bruce E. Cohen, and Robert B. Anderson

13   Free/Turndown Gastrocnemius Flap Augmentation.........   81
     Katarina Nilsson-Helander, Leif Swärd,
     Michael R. Carmont, Nicklas Olsson, and Jon Karlsson

14   Free Hamstring Open Augmentation
     for Delayed Achilles Tendon Rupture....................   85
     Michael R. Carmont, Karin Grävare Silbernagel,
     Katarina Nilsson-Helander, and Jon Karlsson

15   Minimally Invasive Peroneus Brevis Tendon Transfer   89
     Rocco Aicale, Domiziano Tarantino, Francesco Oliva,
     Michael R. Carmont, and Nicola Maffulli

16   Ipsilateral Free Semitendinosus Tendon
     Graft with Interference Screw Fixation   93
     Rocco Aicale, Domiziano Tarantino, Francesco Oliva,
     Michael R. Carmont, and Nicola Maffulli

17   Endoscopic-Assisted Free Graft Technique
     with Semi-T Transfer   99
     Hajo Thermann and Christoph Becher

18   Endoscopic Flexor Hallucis Longus Tendon Transfer........   103
     Michael R. Carmont, Jordi Vega, Jorge Batista,
     and Nuno Corte-Real

Part V   Achilles Tendon Lengthening

19   Minimally Invasive Lengthening of the Achilles Tendon   113
     Olof Westin, Jonathan Reading, Michael R. Carmont,
     and Jon Karlsson

20   Gastrocnemius Slide   119
     Christoph Becher and Hajo Thermann

Part VI   Achilles Tendon Shortening

21   Z Shortening of Healed Achilles Tendon Rupture...........   125
     Rocco Aicale, Domiziano Tarantino, Alessio Giai Via,
     Francesco Oliva, and Nicola Maffulli

22 Endoscopically Assisted Mini-open Technique 129
Hajo Thermann and Christoph Becher

Part VII Biologics in Tendon Healing

23 Biologics in Tendon Healing: PRP/Fibrin/Stem Cells 135
Paul W. Ackermann

Index 147

Part I

Acute Achilles Tendon Ruptures: Suture Techniques

Open Standard Technique

1

Jon Karlsson, Nicklas Olsson, Michael R. Carmont, and Katarina Nilsson-Helander

1.1 Indication and Diagnosis

Acute Achilles tendon rupture usually occurs in the midportion 2–6 cm proximal from the insertion site of calcaneus. In general there are usually no warning symptoms and the injury frequently occurs with a very distinct ankle trauma. The rupture is generally total and partial Achilles tendon rupture is very rare in the cases of specific pop sensed and localized to the midportion of the tendon. The diagnosis is clinical with positive Thompson's test (calf squeeze test), reduced plantar flexion strength, and a palpable gap in the tendon. Surgical and nonsurgical treatment is still debated, together with the timing of the key components of rehabilitation, e.g., weight-bearing, movement, and functional bracing [1]. Open surgery (end-to-end repair) may be considered the gold standard surgical procedure. There has been shown no advantage in a fascial turndown over end-to-end appositional repair for acute ruptures [2]. Primary repair without an augmentation can be performed approximately within 3 weeks. Contraindications include peripheral vascular diseases, skin affections, and systemic diseases with high risk of infection.

1.2 Operative Setup

Open end-to-end repair can be carried out in local, regional, or general anesthesia. The procedure is performed with a patient placed in prone position, with the feet over a pillow or outside the operating table. A setup of excessive plantar flexion increases the risk of overtightening the repair and shortening of the tendon. The risk of lengthening is a more common issue and should be avoided. Tendon lengthening will lead to reduced plantar flexion strength [3]. Therefore it is wise to dress the uninjured side to be able to compare the neutral position. A wedge can be used below the contralateral pelvis to straighten the position of the hind foot. Antibiotic prophylaxis is recommended (local recommendations decides the type of antibiotics) to reduce the risk of the major complication of deep infection. Prophylaxis against deep-vein thrombosis is recommended due to the high risk of deep venous thrombosis [4]. A tourniquet is generally not needed.

J. Karlsson, MD, PhD (✉) • N. Olsson, MD, PhD
K. Nilsson-Helander, MD, PhD
Department of Orthopedics, Sahlgrenska Academy, University of Gothenburg, Gothenburg, Sweden
e-mail: jon.karlsson@telia.com; nicklas.olsson@gu.se; Ina.nilsson@telia.com

M.R. Carmont, FRCS(Tr&Orth)
The Department of Orthopaedic Surgery, Princess Royal Hospital, Shrewsbury & Telford Hospital NHS Trust, Shropshire, UK
e-mail: mcarmont@hotmail.com

© ESSKA 2017
H. Thermann et al. (eds.), *The Achilles Tendon*, DOI 10.1007/978-3-662-54074-9_1

1.3 Surgical Technique

A 5–8 cm posteromedial skin incision is preferred to minimize any risk of injury to the branches of the sural nerve. The paratenon should be carefully identified before further incision to optimize the wound closure (Fig. 1.1). The paratenon is opened centrally and the frayed ends are easily visualized. In general, healthy tendon is located in proximal and distal direction from the rupture site (Fig. 1.2). This is where to place the sutures for greatest stability. The skin and subcutaneous tissue should be handled with care due to the limited blood supply, in order to reduce the risk of tissue breakdown. The gap and tendon ends are cleaned and carefully debrided to optimize the repair. The ends should be apposed without major tension. There are different sutures and techniques in the literature, but this suture technique is the author's preference [5].

A combination of both core and circumferential sutures are used for a stable repair. The core suture consists of two semi-absorbable sutures (No. -2) using a modified Kessler technique [6]. The double Kessler locking loop should be carefully placed away from the rupture site in healthy tendon (Fig. 1.3). The sutures must be able to glide and also care to not damage the core sutures with the needle. The foot is placed in 20–30° plantarflexion when tying the sutures. The uninjured side, tendon quality, and tension are all used to estimate the tendon length. One can also take into account a lengthening of approximately 1 cm until the tendon is healed [7]. Next a running circumferential suture is used with absorbable sutures (No. -0) using an epitendinal crisscross technique described by Silfverskiold et al. to reinforce the core sutures (Fig. 1.4) [8]. The paratenon should be carefully repaired, thereafter using absorbable subcutaneous sutures and meticulous wound closure with nylon sutures.

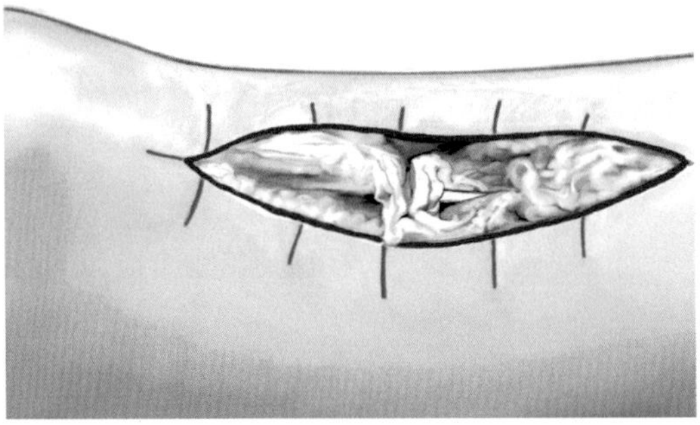

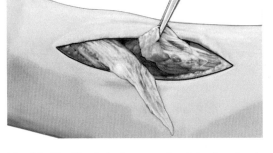

Fig. 1.1 Posteromedial skin incision and identification of paratenon

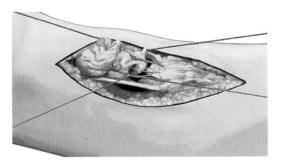

Fig. 1.2 The blood clot is removed and the frayed ends are identified and debrided. Healthy tendon is seen in the distal end

Fig. 1.3 The first core suture is applied in healthy tendon. Both core sutures are in place and tied from each side to the estimated tendon length. A gentle pressure could be applied in ankle dorsal flexion to feel the stability of the sutures and for correct tension in the sutures before tying. The plantaris tendon is visualized in the figure

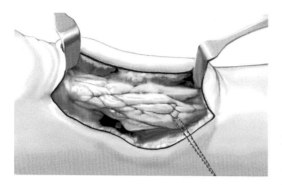

Fig. 1.4 The tendon is sutured in a circumferential criss-cross technique to reinforce the repair

1.4 Postoperative Care

In the first phase of wound healing, a cast is applied for 2 weeks. No weight-bearing is allowed in this stage when the ankle is positioned in plantarflexion. Next, the sutures are removed (day 14), and a pneumatic walker brace with heel pads is adopted. Generally three pads are used and these are gradually removed in 6 weeks. Full weight-bearing is encouraged from the first day with brace. A physical therapist continuously should follow a standardized rehabilitation protocol.

1.5 Pearls Tips and Pitfalls

- Stable surgical technique allows early range of motion training and early weight-bearing.
- The tendon length is probably crucial for the result, but the estimated length is difficult during the surgical repair.

References

1. Khan RJ, Carey Smith RL. Surgical interventions for treating acute Achilles tendon ruptures. Cochrane Database Syst Rev (Online). (2010);(9):CD003674. doi:10.1002/14651858.CD003674.pub4.

2. Heikkinen J, Lantto I, Flinkkila T, Ohtonen P, Pajala A, Siira P, Leppilahti J. Augmented compared with nonaugmented surgical repair after total achilles rupture: results of a prospective randomized trial with thirteen or more years of follow-up. J Bone Joint Surg Am. 2016;98(2):85–92. doi:10.2106/JBJS.O.00496.

3. Silbernagel KG, Steele R, Manal K. Deficits in heel-rise height and Achilles tendon elongation occur in patients recovering from an Achilles tendon rupture. Am J Sports Med. 2012;40:1564–71. doi:10.1177/0363546512447926.

4. Nilsson-Helander K, Thurin A, Karlsson J, Eriksson BI. High incidence of deep venous thrombosis after Achilles tendon rupture: a prospective study. Knee Surg Sports Traumatol Arthrosc. 2009;17(10):1234–8. doi:10.1007/s00167-009-0727-y.

5. Olsson N, Silbernagel KG, Eriksson BI, Sansone M, Brorsson A, Nilsson-Helander K, Karlsson J. Stable surgical repair with accelerated rehabilitation versus nonsurgical treatment for acute achilles tendon ruptures: a randomized controlled study. Am J Sports Med. 2013;41(12):2867–76. doi:10.1177/0363546513503282.

6. Kessler I. The "grasping" technique for tendon repair. Hand. 1973;5(3):253–5.

7. Kangas J, Pajala A, Ohtonen P, Leppilahti J. Achilles tendon elongation after rupture repair: a randomized comparison of 2 postoperative regimens. Am J Sports Med. 2007;35(1):59–64.

8. Silfverskiold KL, Andersson CH. Two new methods of tendon repair: an in vitro evaluation of tensile strength and gap formation. J Hand Surg Am. 1993;18(1):58–65. doi:10.1016/0363-5023(93)90246-Y.

Percutaneous Suturing with a Double-Knot Technique

2

Hajo Thermann and Christoph Becher

2.1 Indication and Diagnosis

Management of Achilles tendon (AT) rupture depends on various factors and can be divided into nonoperative and operative treatment. Many different techniques have been described for operative treatment, with a lack of consensus regarding the best option [1]. For acute rupture, percutaneous repair of the AT is associated with a relatively low complication rate (particularly regarding wound disorders and infection) and high level of patient satisfaction [1, 2]. It was shown that percutaneous repair of the AT resulted in reduced costs and comparable outcome and complications rates to open repair [3]. A further advantage of the presented technique is the remaining integrity of the paratenon, which is essentially important for the healing process.

The best indications for percutaneous AT repair are patients with an acute rupture 2–6 cm proximal to the calcaneal insertion with sono-graphical adaptation of the tendon stumps at plantar flexion. Since percutaneous repair

techniques demonstrated an increased susceptibility to early repair elongation compared with the open technique [4], athletes or patients that warrant accelerated rehabilitation are questionable good candidates for percutaneous repair since the repair should be sufficiently protected postoperatively to allow for biological healing and avoid early repair elongation and potential gapping between the healing tendon ends. The at this point presented technique might overcome these drawbacks due to the possibly increased stiffness of the tape used for augmentation [5] and the double-knot technique.

Distal ruptures <2 cm proximal to the calcaneal insertion need other treatment considerations to maintain end-to-end tendon apposition and suture stability. To avoid suture pull-through, the small distal stump, the internal fixator used for the percutaneous suture, should be passed through a trans-osseous calcaneal tunnel, or a different technique with direct anchoring of the tendon into the calcaneal insertion should be used.

H. Thermann (✉) • C. Becher
International Center of Hip-, Knee- and Foot Surgery,
ATOS Clinic Heidelberg, Heidelberg, Germany
e-mail: thermann@atos.de; becher.chris@web.de

© ESSKA 2017
H. Thermann et al. (eds.), *The Achilles Tendon*, DOI 10.1007/978-3-662-54074-9_2

2.2 Operative Setup

The procedure is performed in the prone position with the leg hanging slightly over the table edge. The other leg is lowered slightly. In order to bring the hindfoot in a straight position, a small wedge is placed below the contralateral pelvis. The lower leg and the foot are in a neutral position. The lower leg can also be stabilized with a gel pad. Care should be paid to prevent pressure damage of the peroneal nerve, the sural nerve, and the foot. A tourniquet can optionally be used with exsanguination of the leg. According to the author's experience, it is recommended to inflate the tourniquet to 300 mmHg. General anesthesia is the most suitable. Antibiotic prophylaxis is recommended by using a third-generation cephalosporin.

The authors use a FiberTape as the internal fixator, which is an ultrahigh strength 2 mm wide tape usable in various situations in ligament or tendon repair (FiberTape®, Arthrex GmbH, München). We recommend after tendon reconstruction to apply fibrin glue (e.g., Tissucol 5 ml) and, if there is the possibility for application, a PRP product, a centrifuge, and appropriate syringe to be available.

2.3 Surgical Technique

Medial and lateral longitudinal incisions just proximal to the insertion of the Achilles tendon and medial next to the rupture site are applied (Fig. 2.1).

The FiberTape is pulled through the tendon from lateral to medial by using a SutureLasso (Arthrex GmbH, München) or an awl directly proximal to the calcaneal insertion of the AT. The FiberTape is then crosswise pulled back to lateral (Fig. 2.2) and again back to medial to have a stronger distal anchorage of the suture (Fig. 2.3).

Both strands are pulled transtendineal through the medial incision at the rupture site (Fig. 2.4).

The two proximal incisions next to the tendon at least 2–3 cm proximal to the rupture site are applied with protection of the sural nerve by a small Hohmann retractor. Then, the lateral strand is pulled out through the proximal lateral incision as well as the medial strand through the medial incision (Fig. 2.5). Tension is applied to the framewise suture to put the foot into equinus position and adapt the tendon ends at the rupture site, which is confirmed by manual palpation. The lateral strand is pulled medially, and a first knot is applied with holding the foot in equinus position (Fig. 2.6).

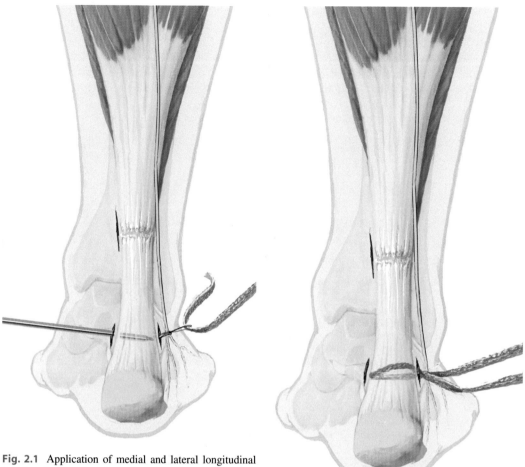

Fig. 2.1 Application of medial and lateral longitudinal incisions just proximal to the insertion of the Achilles tendon and medial next to the rupture site

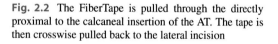

Fig. 2.2 The FiberTape is pulled through the directly proximal to the calcaneal insertion of the AT. The tape is then crosswise pulled back to the lateral incision

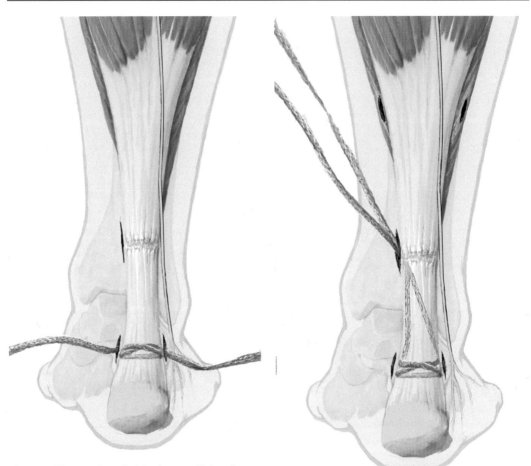

Fig. 2.3 The tape is pulled back to medial to have a stronger distal anchorage of the suture

Fig. 2.4 Both strands of the tape are pulled transtendineal through the medial incision at the rupture site

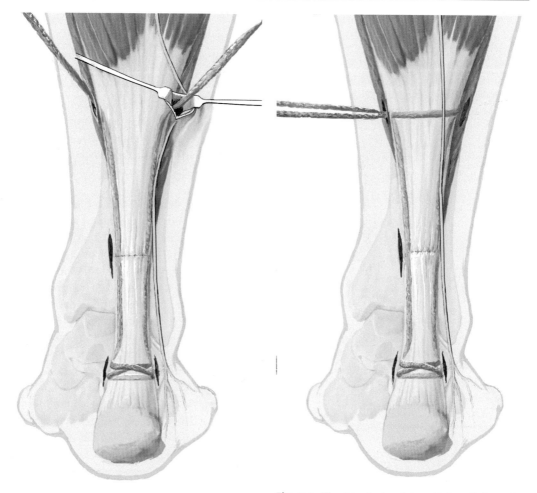

Fig. 2.5 The lateral strand of the tape is pulled out through the proximal lateral incision and the medial strand through the medial incision

Fig. 2.6 The lateral strand is pulled medially and to apply a first knot with holding the foot in equinus position

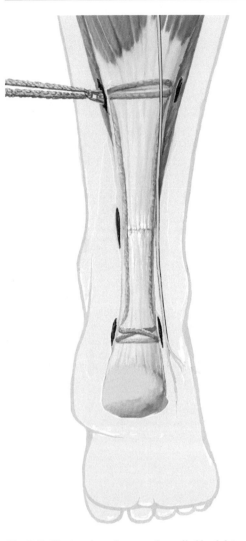

Fig. 2.7 The tape is again crosswise pulled back laterally and medially and knotted again through the proximal medial incision

2.4 Postoperative Care

After application of the wound dressing using cotton wool fixed with an elastic bandage, a prefabricated cardboard splint is applied in equinus position. This device can also be used as a night splint. With good wound and swelling conditions, full weight bearing is allowed in the boot (Vario-Stabil, Orthotech GmbH, 82131 Gauting-Stockdorf) from the second postoperative day.

The Vario-Stabil: It has a plastic tongue to prevent dorsiflexion; the lateral shaft stabilization reduces torsion, and the reducible heel pad allows a gradual adjustment of 20° from plantar flexion to neutral position. With the fitted boot, the patient is allowed to perform full weight bearing and to continue the previously begun isometric exercises. The patient wears the boot for 6 weeks, day and night (or alternatively the night splint to protect the tendon), and for the following 2 weeks, only during the daytime [6].

Plantar flexion exercises are allowed from the beginning. After 3 weeks the patient is allowed to exercise on a stationary bike but only with little application of power. After 4 weeks, a physiotherapeutic treatment is allowed, with well-dosed strengthening exercises (isometric exercises, isokinetic bicycle), proprioceptive neuromuscular facilitation (PNF), and coordination exercises in the boot. In addition, ultrasound application (1 Hz) and cryotherapy are performed to enhance tendon regeneration. From the sixth week on, the leg-press training is begun in the boot. After 8 weeks, an ultrasonographic control evaluates the restoration of the continuity and the tendon regeneration. Achieving an appropriate tendon regeneration (8–12 weeks MRI/sonography control), the treatment in the boot is discontinued. A small heel lift in the normal shoe is recommended for further 6–8 weeks. Jogging is allowed after 3 months if the coordination and muscle power are appropriate.

The tape is again crosswise pulled back laterally and medially and knotted again through the proximal medial incision (Fig. 2.7).

Fibrin glue (e.g., Tissucol 5 ml) and a PRP product are injected under visual control in the rupture site. The application of a drain is not necessary. The incisions are closed in common fashion and the skin infiltrated with a local anesthetic (e.g., bupivacaine 0.5%).

2.5 Pearls, Tips, and Pitfalls

- The knot is applied in 20° of plantar flexion.
- After fixing the first proximal knot, slight plantar flexion and dorsiflexion should be performed to tighten the FiberTape in the aponeurosis; then, the next suture is performed.
- The lateral proximal stab incision should be about 10 mm in length to be able to identify the sural nerve.
- After fibrin glue application, the ankle is moved several times to liberate the tissue adjacent to the repaired tendon from gluing with the tendon which can lead to an anterior scar formation. This "local tightness" in the course of healing could be a source of re-rupture.
- As the construct is stable, mild plantar flexion can be started to prevent the scar formation mentioned above and enhance healing response.

References

1. Khan RJ, Fick D, Keogh A, Crawford J, Brammar T, Parker M. Treatment of acute achilles tendon ruptures. A meta-analysis of randomized, controlled trials. J Bone Joint Surg Am. 2005;87(10):2202–10.
2. McMahon SE, Smith TO, Hing CB. A meta-analysis of randomised controlled trials comparing conventional to minimally invasive approaches for repair of an Achilles tendon rupture. Foot Ankle Surg. 2011;17(4):211–7.
3. Carmont MR, Heaver C, Pradhan A, Mei-Dan O, Gravare SK. Surgical repair of the ruptured Achilles tendon: the cost-effectiveness of open versus percutaneous repair. Knee Surg Sports Traumatol Arthrosc. 2013;21(6):1361–8.
4. Clanton TO, Haytmanek CT, Williams BT, Civitarese DM, Turnbull TL, Massey MB, et al. A biomechanical comparison of an open repair and 3 minimally invasive percutaneous Achilles tendon repair techniques during a simulated, progressive rehabilitation protocol. Am J Sports Med. 2015;43(8):1957–64.
5. Viens NA, Wijdicks CA, Campbell KJ, Laprade RF, Clanton TO. Anterior talofibular ligament ruptures, part 1: biomechanical comparison of augmented Brostrom repair techniques with the intact anterior talofibular ligament. Am J Sports Med. 2014;42(2):405–11.
6. Thermann H. Rupture of the Achilles tendon–conservative functional treatment. Z Orthop Ihre Grenzgeb. 1998;136(5):Oa20–2.

Three-Bundle Technique

Gwendolyn Vuurberg and C. Niek van Dijk

3.1 Indication and Diagnosis

For the diagnosis of an Achilles tendon rupture (Fig. 3.1), it is important to inquire about the patients' history. They may recall a loud 'snapping' sound and a short stab of pain that may be experienced as a kick in the area of the Achilles tendon [3]. On physical examination the course of the Achilles tendon may be visibly and palpably interrupted by indentation. A few hours after the trauma, the gap, however, may be invisible due to swelling and due to a haematoma and oedema. In case of a positive calf squeeze test, a total rupture is indicated [5]. Additional diagnostics may consist of roentgenography (x-ray), ultrasonography (US) and magnetic resonance imaging (MRI). Active patients should be offered both conservative and surgical treatment. Athletes most often are offered the surgical treatment option. It has advantages over conservative treatment, especially in athletes, as it allows early mechanical loading in an accelerated rehabilitation protocol [4]. The three-bundle technique is preferred in the acute situation as the preinjury tendon length can be achieved, allowing re-establishment of maximum isokinetic strength of the Achilles tendon, and can bear a higher load after surgery compared to other techniques like the Krakow locking loop technique [2]. Compared to conservative treatment, immobilization time is reduced, safe early return to weight-bearing is allowed, and risk of re-rupture is diminished [1].

G. Vuurberg • C.N. van Dijk, MD PhD (✉)
Academic Medical Center, Department of
Orthopaedic Surgery G4-264, Meibergdreef 9,
1105 AZ Amsterdam, The Netherlands
e-mail: g.vuurberg@amc.uva.nl;
C.N.vandijk@amc.uva.nl

© ESSKA 2017
H. Thermann et al. (eds.), *The Achilles Tendon*, DOI 10.1007/978-3-662-54074-9_3

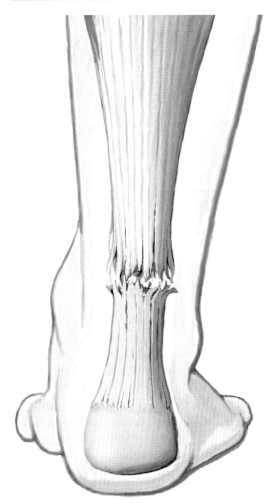

Fig. 3.1 Ankle with torn Achilles tendon

3.2 Operative Setup

For this procedure the patient is placed in a prone position. Support under the lower leg allows free foot movement. The procedure can be performed under general, spinal or combined sciatic-femoral regional block anaesthesia. A bloodless field is not needed. A soft roll or pillow may be placed under the patient's leg to achieve the correct position. This position prevents excessive plantar flexion, to avoid overtightening of the Achilles tendon, and therefore avoids shortening of the tendon and loss of range of motion (ROM). For this reason, the position of the foot should be compared to the position of the other foot in neutral position. The tension of the repair and the balance between dorsi- and plantar flexors should be tested. Standard materials can be used for this technique, including a retractor, a resector and Ethilon 3.0 sutures. After surgery a cast or rigid splint is applied in 20° plantar flexion.

3.3   Surgical Technique

A posteromedial longitudinal approach is used to minimize the risk of injury to the branches of the sural nerve and to preserve the anterior mesotenon. A retractor is used to expose the Achilles tendon. A standard medial incision of 10–12 cm of the skin and tendon sheath is made. Healthy tendon should be exposed at the proximal and distal ends. Care must be taken while handling the skin and subcutaneous tissue to avoid damage to the anterior blood supply of the tendon. For this reason dissection should be minimized. After exposure, the tendon fibres are adapted into three bundles using atraumatic resorbable Vicryl 2 sutures. Bunnell sutures are used to approximate the three bundles while the foot is in maximal plantar flexion (Figs. 3.2, 3.3, 3.4 and 3.5). Subsequently the paratenon and skin are closed using atraumatic sutures.

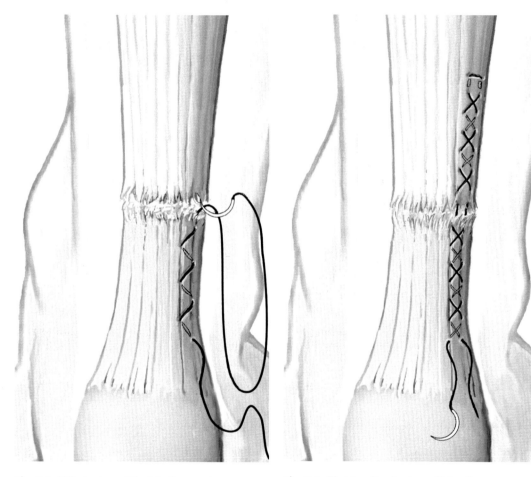

Fig. 3.2 Offset sutures. The thin lines represent sutures inside the tendon

Fig. 3.3 First bundle of sutures. Using the same suture wire in reverse after 6 stitches (3 on each end of the tear)

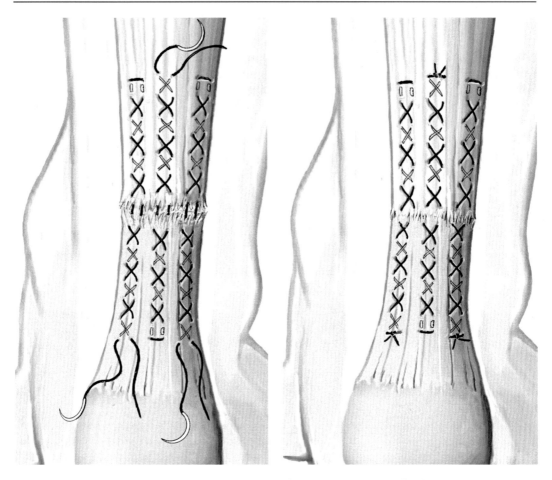

Fig. 3.4 Fully sutured Achilles tendon using 3 bundles of sutures

Fig. 3.5 Sutured tendon after tightening and knotting the sutures

3.4 Postoperative Care

After surgery a lower leg cast is applied in neutral position for 2 weeks. The strength of the sutures leads to elongation at muscular level without deleterious effects on the sutured tendon [6]. Patients are allowed to get out of bed on the first postoperative day, with the help of arm crutches. After 14 days staples/sutures are removed, and the cast is replaced by a functional brace for 4 weeks. For the following 2 weeks, partial weight-bearing is advised, in combination with daily ROM exercises and exercises with a rubber band. From week 4–8, weight-bearing is progressed to full weight-bearing. From week 6, a more intensive programme is commenced focusing on ROM, stretching, proprioception and isometric exercises. After week 8 the boot may be abandoned. Return to work is generally allowed after 60 days. Normal sports activity can be resumed after 5–6 months [1].

3.5 Pearls, Tips and Pitfalls

- A bloodless field is not needed for this procedure.

- Lengthening of the tendon should be avoided at all times as it reduces plantar flexion strength.

References

1. Jaakkola JI, Beskin JL, Griffith LH, Cernansky G. Early ankle motion after triple bundle technique repair vs. casting for acute Achilles tendon rupture. Foot Ankle Int. 2001;22(12):979–84.
2. Jaakkola JI, Hutton WC, Beskin JL, Lee GP. Achilles tendon rupture repair: biomechanical comparison of the triple bundle technique versus the Krakow locking loop technique. Foot Ankle Int. 2000;21(1):14–7.
3. Kerkhoffs GM, Struijs PA, Raaymakers EL, Marti RK. Functional treatment after surgical repair of acute Achilles tendon rupture: wrap vs walking cast. Arch Orthop Trauma Surg. 2002;122(2):102–5.
4. Olsson N, Silbernagel KG, Eriksson BI, Sansone M, Brorsson A, Nilsson-Helander K, Karlsson J. Stable surgical repair with accelerated rehabilitation versus nonsurgical treatment for acute Achilles tendon ruptures: a randomized controlled study. Am J Sports Med. 2013;41(12):2867–76.
5. van der Werken C, Marti RK. Rupture of the Achilles tendon. Ned Tijdschr Geneeskd. 1980;124(32):1321–2.
6. van Dijk CN, Karlsson J, Maffulli N, Thermann H. Open surgery. In: Achilles tendon rupture: current concepts. Surrey: DJO publications; 2008.

Lace Technique Modified by Segesser and Weisskopf

4

Lukas Weisskopf and Anja Hirschmüller

4.1 Indication and Diagnosis

Achilles tendon (AT) ruptures usually occur in sportsmen and physically active individuals with high functional demands, whereby injuries in recreational athletes account for 75% of AT ruptures, 8–20% of the ruptures occur in competitive athletes [1, 2].

Therefore, the goal of any treatment in those athletic individuals is to optimally restore the function of the tendon and the rear foot control. To achieve this goal, the correct length of the Achilles tendon needs to be properly reconstructed, because elongation leads to loss of function [3–6].

It is well known from biomechanical studies that the highest primary pullout force can be achieved by an open Achilles tendon repair, ideally with the triple-bundle technique [3–6], and that conservative therapy has lower plantar flexion strength capacities compared to surgical reconstruction [7, 8].

Additionally, we observed atypical ruptures or multiple stage ruptures in over 10% of our own athletic population. The latter are sometimes very difficult to diagnose (e.g., insertional or proximal lesions) and can only be addressed with an open approach. The "typical," most common, one-stage rupture 4–8 cm above the calcaneal insertion is always asymmetrical. In 80% of all cases, the soleus muscle is separately disconnected from the superficial fibers of the gastrocnemius complex. As the soleus muscle is the main plantar flexor of the AT (especially in knee-flexed position) with a flexion momentum of 40% (gastrocnemius 33%, toe flexors 27%) [3–6, 9], it needs to be pulled and refixed distally to achieve the best functional outcome.

As elongation is in our opinion the most common problem following AT reconstructions, this problem should be properly addressed by a stable suture and an adequate rehabilitation. One main contributor to the high prevalence of elongations may be a too high force acting on the Achilles tendon in the brace/shoe/orthotic device used for functional rehabilitation.

Therefore, since there are often higher biomechanical pullout forces reached by the used suture techniques than protected by the forces in different orthoses, a modified patient rehabilitation protocol and a strong biological and anatomical repair appear necessary for an optimized success of Achilles tendon repair.

L. Weisskopf, MD (✉) • A. Hirschmüller, MD
ALTIUS Swiss Sportmed Center,
Habich-Dietschy-Strasse 5a,
CH -4310 Rheinfelden, Switzerland
e-mail: lukas.weisskopf@altius.ag;
anja.hirschmueller@altius.ag

© ESSKA 2017
H. Thermann et al. (eds.), *The Achilles Tendon*, DOI 10.1007/978-3-662-54074-9_4

4.2   Operative Setup

The operation is performed in prone position with the leg hanging slightly over the table's edge. The contralateral leg is slightly lowered. Great attention should be paid to prevent pressure damage of the peroneal nerve, sural nerve, and the foot. A tourniquet should be used with exsanguination of the leg. It is recommended to inflate the tourniquet to 300 mmHg. General anesthesia is the most suitable anesthesia but not mandatory. Antibiotic prophylaxis is recommended by using a third-generation cephalosporin.

A normal surgical set is composed of a knife, tweezer, scissors, electrocauterization, open tendon stripper, and 6–8 slightly curved, small, sharp-ended clamps. For aftercare, a lower leg splint is applied in plantar flexion.

4.3   Surgical Technique

A medial paraachillar incision about 10 to 12 cm long is applied. Distally the incision has to be curved toward lateral if necessary. The subcutaneous soft tissue is spread with the scissors and the dorsal portion of the Achilles tendon paratenon exposed. Up next the paratenon is splitted, the rupture site is exposed, and the corresponding tendon fibers from the soleus and gastrocnemius are identified (Figs. 4.1 and 4.2). Sometimes asymmetrical and proximalized tendon parts needed to be detected. The plantaris tendon is separated and if still intact cut under slight tension with the open stripper as proximal as possible; the distal attachment stays at the calcaneus. The plantaris tendon is then covered and protected with a wet gauze pad.

First the often isolated disrupted soleus tendon fibers are reattached to the distal stump with a #0 resorbable Vicryl fiber in Mason-Allen technique in maximum plantar flexion position of the foot, which needs to be controlled during the whole surgery. The insertion of the soleus fibers is medial at the calcaneus, medial gastrocnemius goes to distal/lateral, and the lateral gastrocnemius goes to proximal/lateral on the calcaneus insertion (Fig. 4.3).

Anatomically correct, the different tendon bundles are laced together under tension with the small clamps and sutured/fixed with #0 resorbable fibers without excessive compression of the tendon to avoid necrosis (Figs. 4.4 and 4.5).

If present, the plantaris tendon is now augmented to the primary modified triple-bundle tendon repair like an additional frame medially and laterally, as well as ventrally and dorsally if the tendon is long enough. The free end of the plantaris is then spliced to form a layer which is sutured on top of the reconstruction as a gliding structure and subcutaneous protection of adhesions (Figs. 4.6, 4.7, and 4.8).

A Redon drainage is inserted after dilution of the wound. Subcutaneous and skin sutures are applied. Steri-Strips are decreasing the tension of the scar and secure the wound healing.

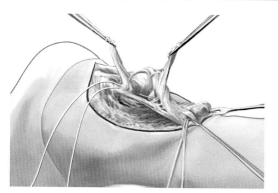

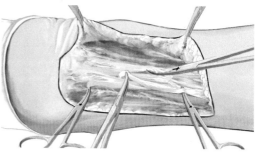

Fig. 4.1 Total Achilles tendon rupture showing typical asymmetrical rupture type with different bundles according the anatomical triple strands (medial/lateral gastrocnemius und soleus)

Fig. 4.4 The bundles were pulled through the corresponding counterpart with small clamps and fix the temporarily refixed

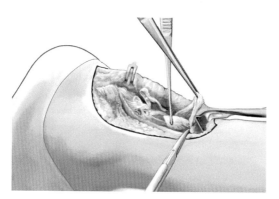

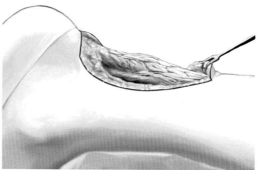

Fig. 4.2 Isolated rupture and disconnected soleus attachment (*right side*)

Fig. 4.5 Completed Achilles tendon reconstruction in lace technique modified by Segesser and Weisskopf in correct tendon length

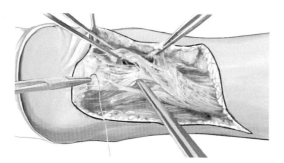

Fig. 4.3 Identification of the different bundles proximally and reconnection to the according anatomical distal part starting with the mostly separated soleus lesion. Remember that the Achilles tendon turns by 90° (soleus to medial calcaneus, medial gastrocnemius to distal/lateral calcaneus, lateral gastrocnemius to proximal lateral calcaneus)

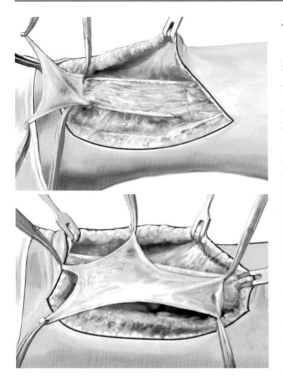

Figs. 4.6 and 4.7 If present, the plantaris tendon is harvested proximally and augmented in a frame type suture technique, first mediolateral and if long enough ventral-dorsally, and fixed with 3-0 resorbable suture

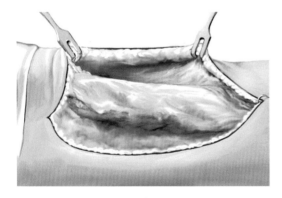

Fig. 4.8 Completed Achilles tendon reconstruction in lace technique modified by Segesser and Weisskopf with plantaris augmentation and reconstruction of a tendon sheet with the spliced end of the plantaris tendon to prevent adhesions

4.4 Postoperative Care

After application of the wound dressing with absorbent cotton, 2 rolls made by compresses are placed beside the wound for reducing the pressure. This is all fixed with an elastic bandage and the foot fixed in plantar flexion by using a lower leg splint. Partial weight bearing with 15 kg for 14 days is recommended to achieve a rapid decongestion. Lymphatic drainage and physiotherapy with motion exercise of the ankle would be beneficial. A stable shoe with 3–4 wedges (3–4 cm) under the heel is given for 6 weeks. Then the shoe is slowly reduced over 4 weeks. Force, endurance, and balance exercises are instructed and cautiously increased.

Running exercises are started after 4 months and competitive sports usually after 6 to 8 months.

4.5 Pearls, Tips, and Pitfalls

- An extensive evaluation of risk factors, especially cortisone injections, nicotine, and others, should be done before indicating an open AR Repair to significantly reduce the risk of wound healing disorders or re-rupture. Note: the risk of wound healing problems after cortisone therapy is up to 56% and re-rupture rate up to 22%.
- Do not strangulate the tendon fibers with the stiches while fixing the strands; otherwise, necrosis areas can be observed.
- If there is only bad or less tissue for the reconstruction and no plantaris tendon for augmentation is present, a gastrocnemius turndown flap can be performed.
- Fix the Achilles tendon in maximal plantar flexion position. There is always the tendency of elongation; they are never too short after the rehabilitation.
- Re-ruptures and elongation occur usually in the first 3 months.
- It is crucial to perform a functional but patiently rehabilitation all the way through controlled by functional testing.

References

1. Leppilahti J, Puranen J, Orava S. Incidence of Achilles tendon rupture. Acta Orthop Scand. 1996;67(3): 277–9.
2. Leppilahti J, Kangas J, Orava S. Achilles tendon ruptures are increasing--surgical or conservative treatment? Duodecim; laaketieteellinen aikakauskirja. 1998;114(2):163–70.
3. Cretnik A, Kosanovic M, Smrkolj V. Percutaneous versus open repair of the ruptured Achilles tendon: a comparative study. Am J Sports Med. 2005;33(9): 1369–79.
4. Cretnik A, Zlajpah L, Smrkolj V, Kosanovic M. The strength of percutaneous methods of repair of the Achilles tendon: a biomechanical study. Med Sci Sports Exerc. 2000;32(1):16–20.
5. Ismail M, Karim A, Shulman R, Amis A, Calder J. The Achillon achilles tendon repair: is it strong enough? Foot Ankle Int. 2008;29(8):808–13.
6. Heitman DE, Ng K, Crivello KM, Gallina J. Biomechanical comparison of the Achillon tendon repair system and the Krackow locking loop technique. Foot Ankle Int. 2011;32(9):879–87.
7. Willits K, Amendola A, Bryant D, Mohtadi NG, Giffin JR, Fowler P, et al. Operative versus nonoperative treatment of acute Achilles tendon ruptures: a multicenter randomized trial using accelerated functional rehabilitation. J Bone Joint Surg Am. 2010; 92(17):2767–75.
8. Lantto I, Heikkinen J, Flinkkila T, Ohtonen P, Siira P, Laine V, et al. A prospective randomized trial comparing surgical and nonsurgical treatments of acute Achilles tendon ruptures. Am J Sports Med. 2016; 44:2406–14.
9. Arndt AN. Entstehung und Auswirkungen asymmetrischer Belastung auf die Achillessehne unter besonderer Berücksichtigung ihrer Morphologie. Dissertation Deutsche Sporthochschule Köln: Sport und Buch Strauß 1997.

Achillon® Achilles Tendon Suture System

5

Andrew J. Roche and James D.F. Calder

5.1 Indication and Diagnosis

Acute, closed rupture of the Achilles tendon can be associated with a classic history of sudden onset of pain with a sense of direct trauma to the Achilles area. Almost always no direct trauma is encountered. It is commonly but not exclusively associated with sporting participation. Early diagnosis is important to ensure the ruptured tendon ends are brought together effectively and protected in an equinus position. Diagnosis can be made by listening to the history and by assessing the patient in the prone position. The injured side has a relatively dorsiflexed ankle position. A gap can frequently be palpated and occassionally seen in the tendon and this may disappear on ankle plantar flexion. Calf squeeze testing may elicit no movement response in ankle plantar flexion. The decision to operate or not has many factors to consider and needs to be carefully discussed with

the patient. Dynamic ultrasound is a useful but not essential imaging modality to aid in surgical planning and the consent process.

The patient must make an informed choice with knowledge of outcomes for both operative and nonoperative interventions including ability to return to work and sports, functional capacity and strength, re-rupture rates and surgical complication rates. Relative surgical indications may include regular or high-level sports participation and a rupture gap of >1 cm between tendon ends that do not appose on ultrasound in the plantar-flexed position. Relative surgical contraindications may include the non-compliant patient, smokers, peripheral vascular disease, diabetics and localised skin lesions. Delayed presentation is not always a contraindication, but the surgeon should consider the need to perform an open repair to appose the tendon ends in injuries presenting more than 4–6 weeks following rupture.

A.J. Roche
The Fortius Clinic, London, UK
e-mail: andy.roche@fortiusclinic.com

J.D.F. Calder (✉)
Consultant Orthopaedic Surgeon, The Fortius Clinic, London, UK

Visiting Professor, Imperial College, London, UK
e-mail: james.calder@fortiusclinic.com

© ESSKA 2017
H. Thermann et al. (eds.), *The Achilles Tendon*, DOI 10.1007/978-3-662-54074-9_5

5.2   Operative Setup

A general anaesthetic is typically used. The patient is positioned in the semi-prone position with the legs positioned prone, the hips semi-prone and the upper body positioned lateral. Minimal bolster support is required. The uppermost forearm is placed in an arm gutter, and a sandbag if desirable can be placed under the uppermost iliac wing to prevent any forward rolling. A tourniquet, if used, is applied around the thigh and inflated to 300 mmHg. It is easiest to apply the tourniquet before the patient is positioned semi-prone. The feet are positioned over the end of the table with padding under both tibiae. It is helpful, but not imperative, to prepare and drape both legs to allow comparison of foot position following tendon repair to ensure appropriate suture tension. Skin sterilisation below the knee is sufficient using an alcoholic chlorhexidine preparation solution. Administration of pre-incision antibiotics as per institution guidance is advised. Potential, but rare, difficulties can be associated with achieving this semi-prone position especially in those with restricted hip external rotation, increased internal tibial torsion or obesity. These patients may, very rarely, be difficult to position with the operating leg prone, in which case a fully prone position may be needed.

5.3   Surgical Technique

The optimal 2–3 cm incision is placed 1 cm below the end of the proximal tendon stump. The incision can feasibly be made horizontally or vertically depending on surgeon preference. The authors have experience of both with no significant complications. The vertical incision, if used, is made just on the medial side of the mid-posterior line. Meticulous skin and tissue handling is imperative throughout this procedure. After the skin is incised, the paratenon, if not already opened as a result of the injury, can be incised (Fig. 5.1). Often a "gap" is seen then with strands of tendon just visible. The tendon ends need to be identified to allow for passage of the Achillon device (Integra LifeSciences Services, Saint Priest, France) (Fig. 5.2). A blunt instrument like a curved, Mayo scissor (or little finger), is useful to penetrate proximally and dissect "around" the tendon end of the proximal stump to ensure it can be mobilised. The procedure is repeated for the distal stump. Whichever tendon stump is approached first (usually the proximal), it is held securely under tension with a soft tissue clamp, and the Achillon device is partially opened with the metal adjustment screw. The device can be widened as required to allow insertion of the central two limbs into the wound on either side of the tendon end stump (Fig. 5.3). Once the device is carefully inserted around the tendon, the sutures are passed through the pre-marked holes in the direction of the arrows (Fig. 5.4). Once all three sutures are passed, the device is carefully withdrawn from the wound allowing the sutures to be retained in the tendon (Fig. 5.5). The three medial and lateral suture ends are simply clamped to the drapes to ensure they do not cross sides. The procedure is repeated for the distal end. It is important that before tying the knots that each suture strand is tested for "reasonable hold" in the tendon by applying a reasonable force on the strand to ensure it does not cut out. If the suture strand cuts out, the suture should be re-inserted by repeating the above steps with the Achillon. The sutures are now ready to be tied typically in a box fashion whilst maintaining the ankle in a plantar-flexed position (Fig. 5.6). Once the knots are tied and cut, the paratenon should be approximated with an absorbable suture to cover the repair. It is usually unnecessary to close the subcutaneous layer separately. The skin is closed with a suture of choice.

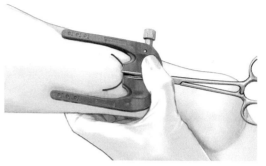

Fig. 5.3 The tendon end is held with the soft tissue clamp as the Achillon is introduced by progressively widening the central limbs using the silver screw

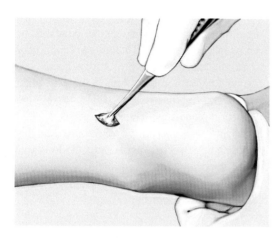

Fig. 5.1 Vertical, slightly medially based incision. The proximal tendon stump is delivered to the wound and held with a soft tissue clamp in preparation for the passage of the Achillon device

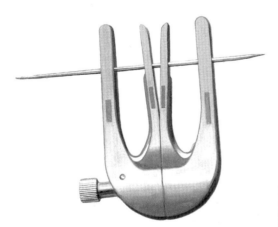

Fig. 5.2 The Achillon device with pre-marked holes to pass the three sutures from one side to the other. The silver adjustment screw opens and closes the two central limbs to allow the tendon stump to fit in between the central limbs during insertion

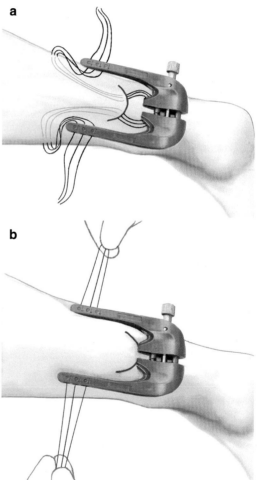

a

b

Fig. 5.4 (**a, b**) The Achillon device central limbs are inserted along the sides of the tendon to allow for passage of the sutures as shown

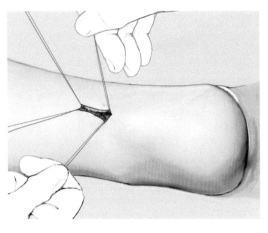

Fig. 5.5 Two sutures placed in both the proximal and distal tendon ends, ready to be tied to in a box fashion to produce a six-strand repair

5.4 Postoperative Care

The ankle is positioned in an equinus plaster slab in 20° to aid skin perfusion for 2 weeks. DVT prophylaxis should be prescribed whilst in the plaster slab. Rest, no weight bearing and elevation should be advised to promote wound healing. From 2 weeks the patient can be placed in a removable boot with heel wedges and encouraged to weight bear with crutches. Active, gentle ankle plantar flexion and dorsiflexion (only to plantigrade) can be started at 3 weeks to minimise paratenon adhesion. The ankle should plantigrade in the boot by 6 weeks and the boot removed by 8 weeks. Passive dorsiflexion should be avoided. A graduated therapy programme should aim for full recovery by around 6 months (this is activity/sports dependent).

5.5 Pearls, Tips and Pitfalls

- To minimise difficulty in the positioning of a patient, the range of hip external rotation and internal tibial torsion should be checked before turning the patient on the table. If necessary, a full prone position may be required (this is very uncommon).
- Placing a pillow under the tibiae can relax the gastrocnemius and make tensioning the repair easier.
- The suture material used is the surgeon's choice. The suture calibre is usually No.2. The authors use No.2 Vicryl or No.2 TiCron™.
- The surgeon must ensure that the suture passed has a good hold on the tendon by applying a reasonable force on each individual suture to ensure it does not cut out.
- To hold the plantar flexion position whilst tensioning, the foot may be placed on the sterile scrub table and the operating table lowered to plantar-flex the ankle if no assistant is available.
- To identify the suture ends to tie together, it can be useful to simply colour code the suture ends with a surgical marker pen to ensure the corresponding and correct proximal and distal limbs are tied together to improve tendon excursion and apposition when tightening the knots.

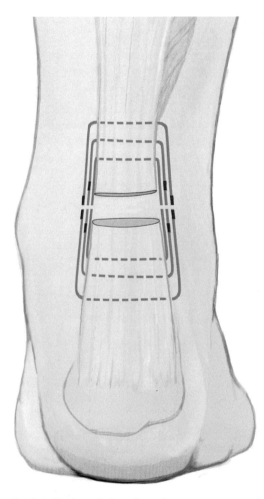

Fig. 5.6 The box stitch configuration

Repair of Distal Achilles Tendon Rupture and Reattachment

6

Michael R. Carmont, Gordon Mackay, and Bill Ribbans

6.1 Indications and Diagnosis

Minimally invasive and percutaneous Achilles tendon repair technique allows direct visualization of end-to-end apposition of the ruptured tendon ends whilst minimizing risks of wound breakdown and infection and improving cosmesis. Although they have these advantages, traditional percutaneous repair techniques have been estimated to have half the strength of open repair methods and also present a risk of iatrogenic sural nerve injury. Biomechanical studies have compared box, Bunnell, modified Bunnell, Kessler and Krackow suture configurations in tendon repair models. The mode of failure of percutaneous repair models is the most commonly suture pull out of the distal Achilles stump, at the tendon suture interface. This leads to the separation of the apposed tendon ends and elongation of the healing tendon. In stronger Krackow sutures, with locking loops, failure tends to occur at the suture knots; however, the insertion of these sutures requires greater access and an open repair.

The Percutaneous Achilles Repair System (PARS) (Arthrex®, Naples, FL) is a jigged device that permits a locking suture to be placed through the tendon after insertion through a small incision at the rupture site. There is no risk of the sural nerve being transfixed, although there is a potential of nerve injury due to needle passage. The sutures can then be preconditioned within the tendon by applying cyclical loading to represent initial weight bearing, before being secured [1]. A large comparison study of a PARS repair and open repairs using Krackow sutures showed no re-rupture in either group. There was however a 2% incidence of suture removal due to foreign body reaction [3].

Although the majority of Achilles tendon ruptures occur at the hypovascular zone 4–6 cm from the insertion, 9% occur more distally (Fig. 6.1), and some "ruptures" are effectively bone avulsions of the tendon from the calcaneum. For distal ruptures, the stump may be so small that it may not be possible to insert sutures securely to permit settling and commence initial loading without risk of suture pull through. To avoid this, the proximal suture ends may be secured by passage through a trans-osseous calcaneal tunnel or by anchoring directly into the bone. Research

M.R. Carmont (✉)
The Department of Orthopaedic Surgery,
Princess Royal Hospital, Shrewsbury & Telford
Hospital NHS Trust, Shropshire, UK
e-mail: mcarmont@hotmail.com

G. Mackay
The Mackay Clinic, Springfield House, Laurel Hill
Business Park, Polmaise Road, Stirling FK7 9JQ, UK
e-mail: gordonmmackay@gmail.com

B. Ribbans
The County Clinic, Northampton,
Nottinghamshire, UK
e-mail: billribbs@uk-doctors.co.uk

© ESSKA 2017
H. Thermann et al. (eds.), *The Achilles Tendon*, DOI 10.1007/978-3-662-54074-9_6

looking at re-rupture rates reported a 6% re-rupture rate in 340 repairs positioned distally through an intra-osseous tunnel [5]. Intra-osseous fixation using a screw also offers the advantage that the repair is knotless and so prominent knots are avoided.

In some cases a sleeve of bone at the insertion site may be avulsed, or reattachment may be required following the excision of a calcified Achilles insertion and an impinging postero-superior calcaneal tubercle [4]. The tendon reattached with direct tendon to bone contact using suture tape and end holding suture locks.

The use of these techniques provides stable distal fixation for distal rupture and avulsions, minimizes or avoids suture pull out and knot prominence and minimizes brace requirements [2].

6.2 Operative Setup

A laminar flow operating theatre is preferable. Popliteal peripheral local anaesthetic nerve blockade or spinal/general anaesthesia rather than field infiltration is required.

The patient is positioned in the recovery position lateral, with the operated side down. The thigh tourniquet should be applied prior to turning. Care must be taken to ensure that the lower shoulder is flexed to prevent arm venous compression. The pelvis is tilted and the operated leg, lower leg, is externally rotated. The opposite hip and knee are flexed, and a supportive strap may be applied around the knee to support the pelvis reducing rotational forces on the lumbar spine.

Two applications of 2% chlorhexidine skin preparation are used up to the tourniquet.

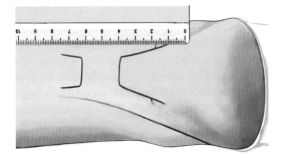

Fig. 6.1 A distal Achilles tendon rupture with only 2 cm of distal stump requiring intra-osseous stabilization

6.3   Surgical Technique

A 2–4 cm incision is made in the midline of the Achilles tendon. The incision is started proximally, just distal to the palpable proximal tendon end and advanced distally. The fascia cruris is then incised longitudinally and the proximal tendon end visualized. The tendon end is then grasped using an Aliss forceps. The branches of the PARS jig are then inserted within the fascia cruris and paratenon layers, although at this level the two layers have usually merged. The predetermined holes on the branches of the jig then allow three sutures to be passed through the tendon (Fig. 6.2). The proximal and distal sutures are transverse, although the middle suture is pulled diagonally through the tendon in the coronal plane using pull-through sutures and around its opposing end, to form a locking loop.

Small longitudinal incisions are then made in the skin over the Achilles insertion, cutting down to bone using a 15 blade. A suture grasper can then be passed either parallel to the tendon or through the substance of the tendon to retrieve the proximal suture from the rupture site. A tip-loaded polyethylene ether ketone (PEEK) suture anchor (4.75 mm) (SwiveLock®, Arthrex, Naples, FL) can then be used to secure the suture into the calcaneum using a drill (3.5 mm), tap, measure and insert sequence with the ankle held in plantar flexion to restore the Achilles Tendon Resting Angle of the non-affected side (Fig. 6.3).

If the trans-osseous technique is used, a 2.5 mm drill is passed across the calcaneum; as the drill is withdrawn, the end of the tunnel is marked using a pen, before the drill tip disappears from sight. A straight 2-0 PDS suture needle is then reversed through the tunnel, holding the sharp end with a clip (Fig. 6.4). The loop allows the sutures from the proximal tendon end to be pulled through the calcaneum (Fig. 6.5). A Mayo needle (PS204B00, Acufirm, Ernst Kratz GmbH) can then be used to pass the suture through the substance of the tendon to the rupture site (Fig. 6.6). The ankle can then be held in plantar flexion and the suture ends tied and buried in the apposed tendon ends in 5–10° of ankle plantar flexion.

For direct reattachment of an avulsed tendon end or reattachment of the Achilles tendon following debridement of a calcified Achilles insertion, the tendon can be reattached directly to bone. Suture tapes, 5 mm (FiberTape®, Arthrex, Naples, FL), can be passed into the tips of two 4.75 mm PEEK suture anchors (SwiveLock®, Arthrex, Naples, FL) and inserted into the proximal site of the Achilles avulsion using the drill, tap and screw insert technique (Fig. 6.7). Both ends of the suture tape can be passed through the proximal portion of the reattachment zone. The ends are then separated, and one from each is crossed and paired with a tape from the other anchor and loaded into third and fourth distal suture anchors. The crossed tapes form an X, and the straight tapes form an II to hold the tendon flat against the avulsed or debrided bone surface (Fig. 6.8). Loose tape and suture ends can then be cut using a scalpel so that there are no prominent knots.

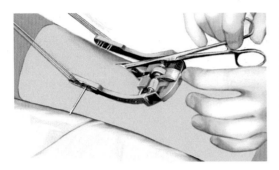

Fig. 6.2 Percutaneous suture is passed through the skin, fascia and the PARS jig

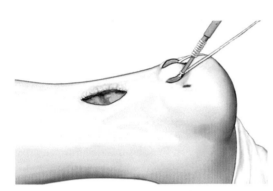

Fig. 6.3 SwiveLock suture anchors for a knotless intra-osseous repair

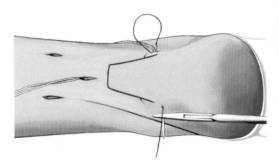

Fig. 6.4 A 2-0 Nylon-straight needle is reversed through the trans-osseous tunnel to act as a pull-through suture

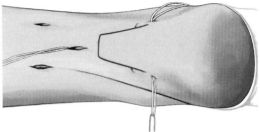

Fig. 6.5 A 2.5 mm drill hole is recommended to allow the passage of three Number 2 strands doubled over

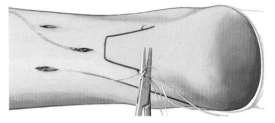

Fig. 6.6 A Mayo needle is used to pass the suture into the repair zone for intra-tendinous suture placement

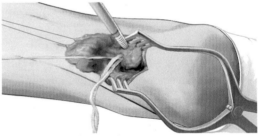

Fig. 6.7 The Fibertape is secured into the calcaneum using a 3.5 mm drill, tap and a 4.75 suture anchor

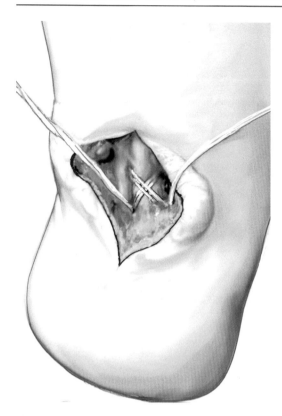

Fig. 6.8 Overall four suture anchors are used with an X and II formation of Fibertapes, holding the tendon flat against the underlying cancellous bone

6.4   Postoperative Care

Postoperatively the patient is placed into a functional brace made from synthetic cast material in equinus or a below knee plaster shell. Once the wound has healed, sutures are removed.

The patient mobilizes toe touch progressing to full weight bearing on the metatarsal heads using axillary crutches as tolerated by pain. Low-molecular-weight heparin is administered for this period. After 2 weeks elbow crutches may be used, and a functional brace with a heel-rise is worn for at-risk activities.

At the 6 weeks time point, the brace is discontinued, and full weight bearing commenced using a 15 mm heel wedge in the shoe on both feet until the 3 months time point.

Formal physiotherapy is commenced with exercises designed to progressively increase the strength and range of motion of the ankle joint. Initially the bilateral standing or seated heel-rises can be initiated to strengthening the calf musculature. The movement should be slow and controlled and both concentric and eccentric contractions should be performed. The load on the injured leg is progressively increased, and the goal is to be able to achieve a unilateral heel-rise in standing.

Other impairments in the lower extremity should also be addressed, and the aim is for the patient to walk without a limp and have normal push off during gait within the first 3–5 weeks. Local massage can reduce adhesions and swelling. Stretching should be avoided and plyometric exercises should only be permitted at the 3 months time point.

No other time guides are recommended after 3 months, and activities including running and jumping can be introduced when the patient has achieved the ability to perform single-leg heel-rises, can walk without a limb and has good single-leg balance.

6.5 Pearls, Tips and Pitfalls

- Stabilizing the end-to-end repair with reduced tendon length with an absolute Achilles Tendon Resting Angle/plantar flexion of +5–10°, to compensate for further suture settling during initial weight bearing.
- Although it may be tempting to try to use a 2 mm drill to form the trans-osseous calcaneal tunnel, the use of a 2.5 mm drill is better. Not only does the surgeon have to pass a needle into a small tunnel entrance aperture, but the passed suture consists of three strands of Number 2 suture which is doubled over for passage.
- The suture anchors can be difficult to insert into a 3.5 mm drill hole even after taping, and a small tap with a mallet may be required to ease insertion.
- Closure of the fascia cruris is essential, this buries any suture knots and restores the tension to the vasculature of both the paratenon and the skin.

References

1. Clanton TO, Haytmanek CT, Williams BT, Civitarese DM, Turnbull TL, Massey MS, Wijdicks CA, LaPrade RF. A biomechanical comparison of an open repair and 3 minimally invasive percutaneous Achilles tendon repair techniques during simulated progressive rehabilitation protocol. Am J Sports Med. 2015; 43(8):1957–64.
2. Groetelaers RPTGC, Janssen L, van der Velden J, Wieland AWJ, Amendt AGFM, Geelen PHJ, Janzing HMJ. Functional treatment or cast immobilization after minimally invasive repair of an acute Achilles tendon rupture: prospective randomized trial. Foot Ankle Int. 2014;35(8):771–8.
3. Hsu AR, Jones CP, Cohen BE, Davis WH, Ellington JK, Anderson RB. Clinical outcomes and complications of percutaneous Achilles repair system versus open technique for acute Achilles tendon ruptures. Foot Ankle Int. 2015;36(11):1279–86.
4. Huh J, Easley ME, Nunley JA. Characterization and surgical management of Achilles tendon sleeve avulsions. Foot Ankle Int. 2016;37(6):596–604.
5. Metz R, van der Heijden GJ, Verleisdonk EJ, Tamminga R, van der Werken C. Persistent disability despite sufficient calf muscle strength after re-rupture of surgically treated acute Achilles tendon ruptures. Foot Ankle Spec. 2011;4(2):77–81.

Part II

Mid Portion Tendinopathy

Open Debridement of Mid-Portion Achilles Tendinopathy

7

Katarina Nilsson-Helander, Nicklas Olsson,
Olof Westin, Michael R. Carmont,
and Jon Karlsson

7.1 Indication and Diagnosis

Achilles tendinopathy, defined as the occurrence of pain, swelling and impaired performance, has incidence 0.2% in the general population. However, the incidence is much higher in recreational runners (9%).

The pathology features an early short-lived initial phase of an inflammatory cellular reaction, progressing to a stage of fibrous tissue proliferation. Ongoing stimuli lead to an imbalance of matrix synthesis and degeneration causing the tendon to become thickened and tender. Intratendinous lesions form as a result of the ongoing degenerative and degradative processes and uncommonly may ultimately calcify [1]. In non-rupture-related surgical treatment of the Achilles tendon, the relative proportion of the tendinosis has increased more than fourfold, from 4% to 21%, over the last 40 years [2]. The most common location is the hypovascular area approximately 2–6 cm proximal to the Achilles insertion to the calcaneus. Etiological factors include overuse and a lack of flexibility, genetic, gender, endocrine and metabolic factors, together with a high BMI [1].

Nonoperative treatment includes rest, activity and training modification and specific loading exercise regimes. Other alternatives, with limited scientific evidence, such as massage therapy, NSAIDs, high-volume and sclerosant injections and in some cases the use of extracorporeal shock wave therapy are used. These can either be alone or in combination. Approximately 25% of patients have persistent symptoms despite prolonged and well-supervised nonoperative therapy, and then surgery can be indicated.

Surgery allows abnormal tissue in the tendon and paratenon to be removed together with disruption of the neovascular tissues and associated nerve fibres. It also has the potential additional benefit of reactivating the healing process. Minimally invasive and endoscopic surgery has the advantage of minimising wound problems [2, 3], although there is a learning curve compared to open surgery. Open surgical technique is relatively simple, allows the possibility of debridement of intratendinous lesions and permits standard reconstructive techniques.

K. Nilsson-Helander • N. Olsson • O. Westin
J. Karlsson (✉)
The Department of Orthopaedic Surgery,
Sahlgrenska Academy, University of Gothenburg,
Gothenburg, Sweden

Department of Orthopaedic Surgery, Kungsbacka
Hospital, Kungsbacka, Sweden
e-mail: Ina.nilsson@telia.com; nicklas.olsson@gu.se;
olof.westin@vgregion.se; Jon.Karlsson@telia.com

M.R. Carmont
The Department of Orthopaedic Surgery,
Princess Royal Hospital, Shrewsbury, UK

Telford Hospital NHS Trust, Shropshire, UK
e-mail: mcarmont@hotmail.com

© ESSKA 2017
H. Thermann et al. (eds.), *The Achilles Tendon*, DOI 10.1007/978-3-662-54074-9_7

Meta-analyses have reported a mean success rate of approximately 85% for surgical procedures for mid-substance tendinosis, with 78% of patients being satisfied by treatment [3, 4]. Physical activity is fully restored in 67% of patients and 83% are asymptomatic. The complication rate has been reported to be as high as 15%, including major complications such as tendon rupture and wound necrosis and minor complications such as superficial infection. Contraindications to open surgery include those with diabetes, heavy smokers and patients with compromised immune systems and peripheral vascular disease.

7.2   Operative Setup

A laminar flow operating theatre is preferable. The patient may be positioned supine with the leg either in the figure-of-4 position or the lateral recovery position with the affected side down with the hip in external rotation, allowing good posteromedial access. A thigh tourniquet should be applied prior to positioning. The use of prophylactic antibiotics is according to the individual surgeon's protocol.

7.3   Surgical Technique

A medial longitudinal incision, adequate to debride the length of tendinopathic area, is performed, typically 5–10 cm long (Fig. 7.1). This is commenced distally to the thickened Achilles tendon and extended proximally. The incision may be made on the medial side of the tendon to permit easy debridement and release of the plantaris tendon and to avoid injury to the sural nerve. Care should be taken to avoid undermining the skin edges.

The fascia cruris and the underlying paratenon are incised to expose the underlying Achilles tendon. The sural nerve passes superficial to the fascia cruris but crosses the lateral border of the Achilles tendon at 8–10 cm from the Achilles insertion to the calcaneus. Using a medial incision, the exposed area is well away from the course of the sural nerve. Iatrogenic injury is unlikely during debridement provided this occurs in a subfascial plane.

The tendon is cleared of any adhesions and thickened layers of paratenon on the dorsal aspect and neovascularisation areas on the ventral side (Figs. 7.2, 7.3, and 7.4). Longitudinal tenotomies are then performed through the thickened section of tendon, taking care to perform the tenotomies parallel with the spiralling tendon fascicles (Fig. 7.5). The tendinopathic tendon is by definition thickened and usually can accommodate up to three tenotomies. The internal architecture of the tendon should be inspected for areas of tendinosis (Fig. 7.6). If macroscopic lesions are present, these should be removed. If less than 50% of the tendon is remaining, reconstruction or augmentation should be considered.

The fascia cruris and paratenon are then closed using detensioning mattress sutures. The wound is carefully closed aiming for low tension at the skin edges. In addition detensioning subcutaneous and skin mattress sutures are applied (Fig. 7.7).

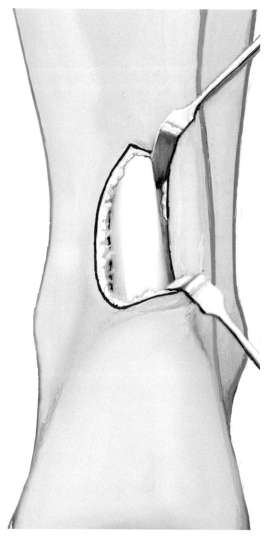

Fig. 7.1 A medial longitudinal incision, adequate to debride the length of tendinopathic tendon is performed, typically 5–10 cm long

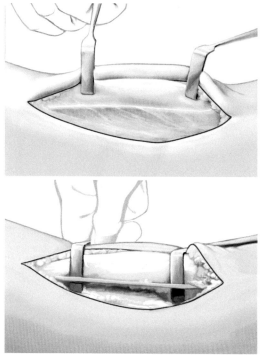

Figs. 7.2 and 7.3 The ventral aspect of the Achilles tendon should be exposed and cleared of thickened neovascular tissue including a release of the plantaris tendon

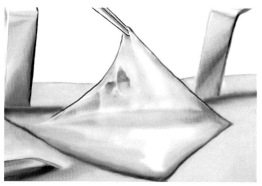

Fig. 7.4 The thickened paratenon should be stripped off the tendinopathic tendon

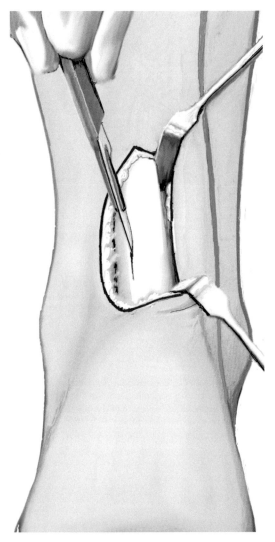

Fig. 7.5 Longitudinal tenotomies parallel with the spiralling tendon fascicles are then performed through the tendon

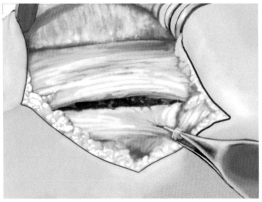

Fig. 7.6 The internal architecture of the tendon should be inspected for areas of tendinosis and any macroscopic lesions should be removed

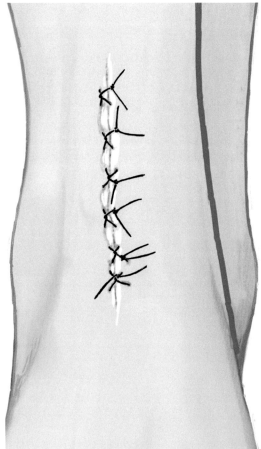

Fig. 7.7 Detensioning mattress sutures should be applied to the subcutaneous tissues and skin

7.4   Post-operative Care

A wound dressing is applied, or a negative pressure dressing may be beneficial in patients with comorbidities. Undercast padding and crepe suffice for immobilisation. In cases where tendon debridement has been performed, a protective anterior plaster of Paris shell may be worn to protect against excessive forceful plantar flexion and dorsiflexion and yet permits early weight bearing, during the first 2 weeks. Weight bearing is permitted as tolerated from the day of surgery.

Early movement is recommended once the wound has healed although sutures should remain in place for up to the 3-week time point to minimise the risks of wound breakdown.

All patients are recommended to follow a symptom and function criterion-based rehabilitation protocol supervised by a physiotherapist twice a week. Patients should start strength training of the gastrocnemius/soleus complex; initially, eccentric loading exercises are commenced, and as tolerated strength and intensity were successively increased. Two-legged heel raises are started as soon as possible depending upon the muscle strength, and ROM was increased.

7.5   Pearls Tips and Pitfalls

- Patients should be made aware of the risks of open Achilles surgery, particularly with respect to wound healing.
- Perpendicular incisions should be made down to the fascia cruris and paratenon.
- Care should be taken to close the paratenon, fascia cruris and skin with detensioning sutures.

References

1. Roche AJ, Calder JDF. Achilles tendinopathy: a review of the current concepts of treatment. Bone Joint J. 2013;95-B:1298–307.
2. Johansson K, Lempainen L, Sarimo J, Laitala-Leinonene T, Orava S. Macroscopic anomalies and pathological findings in and around the Achilles tendon. Observations from 1661 operations during a 40 years period. Orthop J Sports Med. 2016;2(12). doi:10.1177/2325967114562371.
3. Lohrer H, David S, Nauck T. Surgical treatment for Achilles tendinopathy- a systematic review. BMC Musculoskeletal Disorders. 2016;17:207.
4. Batles TPA, Zwiers R, Wiegerinck JI, Van Dijk CN. Surgical treatment for midportion Achilles tendinopathy: a systematic review. Knee Surg Sports Traumatol Arthrosc. 2016. [epub ahead of print].

Endoscopic Debridement

8

Hajo Thermann and Christoph Becher

8.1 Indication and Diagnosis

Painful, palpable thickening of the mid-portion of the Achilles tendon, about 2–8 cm proximal to the insertion at the calcaneus, is typically found in mid-portion Achilles tendon tendinopathy. Most patients with chronic painful mid-portion Achilles tendinopathy can be treated conservatively with good outcomes.

Surgery is indicated in symptomatic patients unresponsive to conservative treatment for at least 3 months, depending on the degenerative changes in the Achilles tendon. The differential diagnosis of chronic dysfunction is between mid-portion tendinopathy and chronic rupture. The ability to perform a one-legged heel rise may help discriminate and is usually possible but painful in mid-portion tendinopathy but impossible with dysfunction related to chronic rupture.

The traditional open surgical treatment of chronic painful mid-portion Achilles tendinopathy has consisted of a dorsal approach for many years with a central longitudinal tenotomy and excision of the degenerated tendon tissue [1]. However, postoperative complication rates have been reported to be high and varying from 4.7 to 11.6% [2]. The endoscopic surgical debridement of the area with the increased vascularization (neovessels and nerves outside the ventral tendon) showed to produce satisfactory clinical results in the short-term and minimized postoperative complications [2]. Contraindications include peripheral vascular disease; otherwise, all mid-portion tendinopathies can be handled endoscopically with appropriate expertise. With chronic rupture additional techniques have to be used.

H. Thermann (✉) • C. Becher
International Center of Hip-, Knee- and Foot Surgery,
ATOS Clinic Heidelberg, Heidelberg, Germany
e-mail: thermann@atos.de; becher.chris@web.de

© ESSKA 2017
H. Thermann et al. (eds.), *The Achilles Tendon*, DOI 10.1007/978-3-662-54074-9_8

8.2   Operative Setup

For the treatment of the mid-portion tendinopathy, standard arthroscopic instruments are used. All endoscopic procedures of the Achilles tendon are performed in the prone position with the leg hanging slightly over the table edge. The other leg is lowered slightly. In order to bring the hindfoot in a straight position, a small wedge is placed below the contralateral pelvis. The lower leg and the foot are in a neutral position. The lower leg can also be stabilized with a gel pad. Care should be paid to prevent pressure damage of the peroneal nerve, the sural nerve and the foot. A tourniquet should be used with exsanguination of the leg. According to the author's experience, it is recommended to inflate the tourniquet to 300 mmHg. General anaesthesia is the most suitable. Antibiotic prophylaxis is recommended by using a third-generation cephalosporin.

An arthroscopy set with a 4.0-mm 30 ° arthroscope is recommended. Additional tools including a 3.8-mm and 5.0-mm shaver, a retro knife (ENT instrument), an electrocauterization hook and a fibrin glue (Tissucol 5 ml) should be available. For the application of a PRP product, a centrifuge and appropriate syringe should be available. For postoperative care, a lower leg splint or a prefabricated cardboard splint is applied in plantar flexion.

8.3   Surgical Technique

A medial incision 1 cm proximal to the insertion of the Achilles tendon is applied for insertion of the arthroscope. A second incision is made at the junction of the tendon and the aponeurosis (Fig. 8.1). The subcutaneous soft tissue is dissected with a mosquito clamp along the dorsal portion of the tendon to create a space for endoscopy (Fig. 8.2). Care must be taken not to go too deep anteriorly, as this may result in the injury of the fascia with potential injury of the neurovascular bundle. The manipulation dorsally and ventrally is carried out from both the proximal and the distal incision. The arthroscope is inserted through the proximal incision, a 3.8-mm shaver from the distal incision (Fig. 8.3). By triangulation, the shaver is brought directly into the surgical field. The arthroscope is slightly tilted anteriorly (Fig. 8.4).

After the Achilles tendon is clearly identified, a cautious and slow resection of the paratenon, neovessels and nerves is carried out with the shaver (Figs. 8.5 and 8.6). This is done carefully and in a stepwise approach, starting in the distal portion. With a better view, the shaver can be changed to a full-radius aggressive 5-mm shaver. Extreme care should be taken when working laterally because of the side branch of the fibular nerve as well as the nearby sural nerve, which is not anterior but posterior. The dorsal portion of the Achilles tendon is usually under pressure due to the increased volume through the degenerative changes. The portals are changed as needed.

In accordance with the MRI findings, a small retro knife is used to make an incision into the degenerative foci, which are shaved in a stepwise fashion. In case of extensive intratendinous degenerative changes (xanthochrome degeneration, vascularization, etc.), the pathological tissue has to be completely debrided. A PRP product is injected under visual control intratendineally after the debridement is completed. During the procedure, haemostasis with electrocauterization has to be gradually performed only in short intervals to prevent heat necrosis due to the increase of the fluid temperature. A drain should be introduced and the incisions are closed in a common fashion.

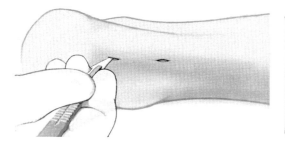

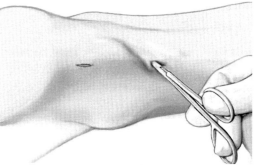

Fig. 8.1 Implementation of the medial incisions; proximal and distal incisions medial to the Achilles tendon. The distal incision has to be proximal to the calcaneal insertion

Fig. 8.2 Mobilization of subcutaneous layer dorsally with a mosquito clamp. Ventral mobilization directly at the Achilles tendon

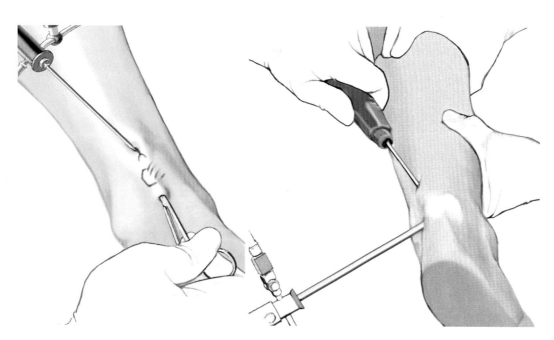

Figs. 8.3 and 8.4 Insertion of the arthroscope from proximal incision and the shaver through the distal incision. The calcaneus is everted in order to operate distally more easily. Optics and shaver meet in a triangulation form

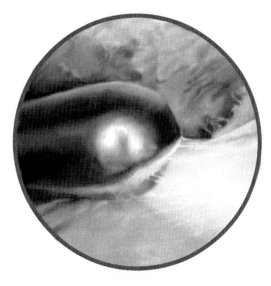

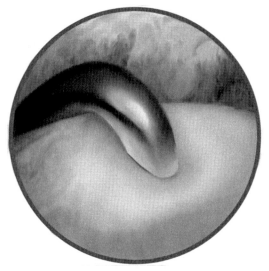

Fig. 8.5 Shaving along the Achilles tendon, the neovascularization in the ventral lying fat tissue until the tendon is completely free. Then, debridement of the peritendineum anteriorly and posteriorly

Fig. 8.6 Incision into the degenerative foci of the tendon with a small retro knife for further debridement

8.4 Postoperative Care

After application of the wound dressing with cotton wool fixed with an elastic bandage, a prefabricated cardboard splint is applied. Movement exercises in dorsiflexion and plantar flexion can start from the second day as tolerated by pain and swelling. We recommend partial weight bearing with 15 kg for 14 days to achieve a rapid decongestion. Lymphatic drainage and physiotherapy with motion exercises of the ankle, especially stretching the flexor chain, are added. After 14 days, full weight bearing is allowed with the use of well-cushioned shoes.

8.5 Pearls Tips and Pitfalls

- Eversion of the calcaneus allows easy handling of the scope and the shaver.
- As the water pressure and the direct contact may lead to irritation of the anterior neurovascular bundle, the fascia should never be opened anteriorly.

- In cases of adhesions or scar formation at the skin, the dorsal space can be widened with a small scissor with careful cuts anteriorly in the direction of the Achilles tendon.
- Along the distal lateral part, there is a small branch of the peroneal artery. After debridement, electrocauterization should be performed under arthroscopical visualization.
- In the proximal medial area, there are small branches of the saphenous vein. Shaving must be performed carefully when reaching the soleus muscle proximally to avoid excess bleeding leading to haematoma formation.

References

1. Alfredson H, Lorentzon R. Chronic Achilles tendinosis: recommendations for treatment and prevention. Sports Med. 2000;29:135–46.
2. Thermann H, Benetos IS, Panelli C, Gavriilidis I, Feil S. Endoscopic treatment of chronic mid-portion Achilles tendinopathy: novel technique with short-term results. Knee Surg Sports Traumatol Arthrosc. 2009;17:1264–9.

Part III

Insertional Tendinopathy

Open Technique

9

Lukas Weisskopf, Patric Scheidegger, Th. Hesse,
H. Ott, and A. Hirschmüller

9.1 Indication and Diagnosis

Noncalcified insertional tendinosis is classified as a painful and usually thickened Achilles tendon insertion up to 2 cm proximal to the calcaneal insertion. It can arise from either an insertional calcification, tendinopathy, partial rupture, or an irritation of the bursa (bursitis calcanea or subachillea) (Fig. 9.1).

It is recommended to conduct an X-ray in the sagittal plane to ensure that no intratendinous calcifications or Haglund exostosis is present. Furthermore, a sonography should be performed to rule out a bursitis subachillea, insertional calcifications (acoustical shadow), partial ruptures, and neovascularization (by Doppler sonography).

The gold standard to determine the quality of the tendon is the MRI with intravenous contrast medium. It enables to exclude partial ruptures or bone edemas, which appear due to friction between the tendon and the calcaneus. Sometimes, intratendinous calcification can be hard to detect in the MRI, and additional imaging is necessary (X-ray or sonography).

Dynamic clinic testing for hindfoot instability is crucial – not only for the diagnosis but also for the treatment. Through this testing malalignments such as increased pronation (pes valgus, pes planus, incorrect footwear) or ankle injuries (chronic ligament injuries) can be detected, and adjustments can be made, for example, by orthopaedic arch support (insoles).

Very important as well is functional analysis to determine possible asymmetrical loading of the Achilles tendon insertion and the hindfoot, e.g., kinematic and kinetic gait and/or running analysis, stabilometry, and isokinetic force testing. If any mechanical cause for the hindfoot instability is not addressed, the success of the therapy options is diminished.

In addition, it is recommended to evaluate for metabolic diseases, especially rheumatic diseases or hyperuricemia.

Frequently, some of the following pathologies can occur in combination. They need to be excluded or diagnosed:

L. Weisskopf (✉) • P. Scheidegger • T. Hesse
H. Ott • A. Hirschmüller
ALTIUS Swiss Sportmed Center,
Habich-Dietschy-Strasse 5a, CH-4310 Rheinfelden,
Switzerland
e-mail: lukas.weisskopf@altius.ag;
patric.scheidegger@altius.ag; thomas.hesse@altius.ag;
henning.ott@altius.ag; anja.hirschmueller@altius.ag

© ESSKA 2017
H. Thermann et al. (eds.), *The Achilles Tendon*, DOI 10.1007/978-3-662-54074-9_9

- Bursitis subachillea
- Bursitis calcanea
- Partial rupture of the Achilles tendon
- Hypertrophy of the processus posterior calcanei
- Intratendinous ossifications
- Morbus Sever (apophysitis calcanei)
- Bone bruise/stress fracture of the calcaneus
- Impingement of the os trigonum
- Entrapment of Ramus calcanearis of the tibial or sural nerve
- Plantar fasciitis
- Instability of the ankle

The typical combination is insertional tendinopathy with partial rupture of the insertion (commonly the deep, ventral part) with Haglund exostosis and bursitis subachillea due to rear foot instability.

As a first therapy option, the conservative treatment should be discussed, especially if a noncalcified situation or no significant partial tear (less than 30%) is present. During this treatment eccentric training with maximal dorsal extension to 0 °, dynamic stability training, high-dose shock wave therapy, as well as orthopedic arch support should be performed. Injection therapies such as sclerotherapy of neovessels or treatment with homeopathic solutions should be evaluated. Steroids are not recommended at all times, because of the danger of severe side effects. Should all these treatments do not lead to a satisfactory outcome, an operative treatment becomes necessary.

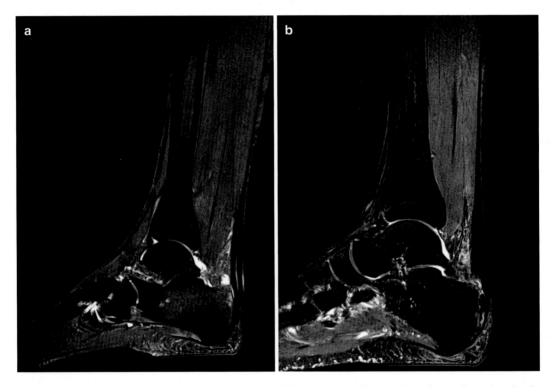

Fig. 9.1 Sagittal MRIs of patients with insertional tendinopathy. *On the left*, (**a**) example of a bursitis subachillea with an edematous irritation of the calcaneus (pronounced Haglund exostosis) and signs of a tendinopathy. *On the right*, (**b**) tendinopathy with typical partial rupture distally and edematous irritation of the calcaneus

9.2   Operative Setup

The operation is performed in the prone position with the foot hanging slightly over the edge of the table. The other leg is slightly lowered. Attention should be paid to prevent any pressure damage of the peroneal nerve, the sural nerve, and the vulnerable skin. A tourniquet inflated to 300 mmHg should be used to prevent exsanguination of the leg. Spinal as well as general anesthesia is suitable. Antibiotic prophylaxis can be considered by using a third-generation cephalosporin.

A common surgical set with a knife, tweezers, scissors, electrocoagulation device, hammer, different sizes of chisels and a pestle, blunt hooks, and bone wax is sufficient for the procedure. For aftercare, a lower leg splint is applied in plantar flexion.

9.3   Surgical Technique

A medial paraachillar incision is made at the ventral border of the Achilles tendon about 4 cm proximal of the thickening. Distally, the incision is curved toward lateral into the transverse skinfolds. Any unnecessary stress or pressure to the skin should be avoided as the risk of wound healing disorders is up to 10% after Achilles tendon insertion procedures. The subcutaneous soft tissue is spread with the scissors to expose the bursa calcanea and the dorsal portion of the Achilles tendon (paratenon) (Fig. 9.2). Up next, the bursa (if inflamed) and the peritendineum are removed. The Achilles tendon is now split in the direction of the fibers, which is not in a straight longitudinal direction (Fig. 9.3). The intratendinous changes are resected elliptically, especially partial ruptures or ossifications (Fig. 9.4). Underneath a potential bursitis, subachillea is excised. If a Haglund exostosis is present and might be the cause of the tendinopathy, it has to be resected and remodeled with a chisel (Fig. 9.5). It is recommended not to resect too much of the calcaneus. Otherwise, the function as a lever arm of the calcaneus will be impaired. Afterward, the surface of the calcaneus should be smoothened with hammer and pestle. To prevent adherence of the Achilles tendon with the cranial surface of the calcaneus, a thin layer of bone wax is applied to the resected zone. The tendon is readapted by using a 2-0 absorbable suture (Fig. 9.6). It is crucial to not put too much tension to the sutures since the tendon fibers might be strangulated otherwise. If more than 60–70% of the insertion is resected, a fixation with transosseous sutures or titanium bone anchor is necessary. Finally, a drain should be introduced and the incisions are closed in a common fashion. We recommend using Steri-Strips to distribute the tension over the suture.

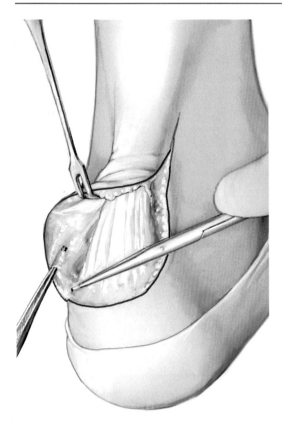

Fig. 9.2 The incision is performed medially and distally curved toward lateral. The dorsal portion of the Achilles tendon is exposed

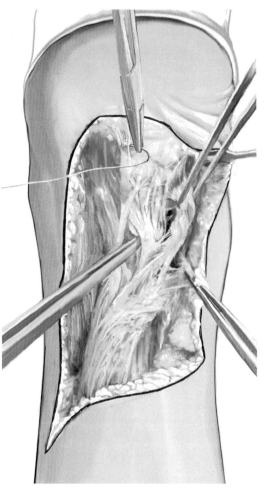

Fig. 9.3 Splitting of the Achilles tendon in the direction of the fibers

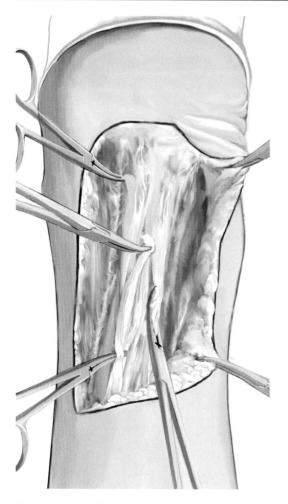

Fig. 9.4 Intratendinous changes (e.g., partial ruptures) have to be resected

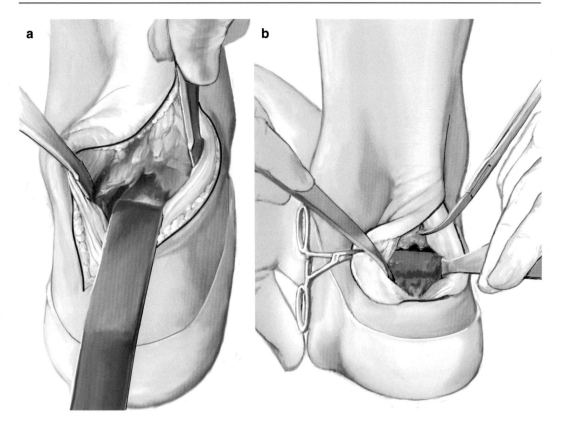

Fig. 9.5 (**a, b**) Resection of a Haglund exostosis with a chisel (**a**). The resected surface should be smoothened with hammer and pestle (**b**)

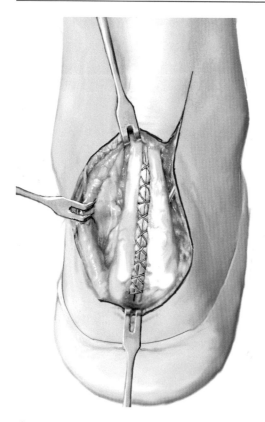

Fig. 9.6 Stitching of the tendon

9.4 Postoperative Care

After application of the wound dressing with an absorbent dressing, two small rolls made by compresses are placed beside the Achilles tendon and fixed with an elastic bandage. It is important to place the foot in plantar flexion by using a lower leg ventral splint during the night.

Partial weight bearing with 15 kg for 10–14 days in the ankle-high rehab shoe is recommended to achieve a rapid decongestion and to support wound healing. Furthermore, lymphatic drainage and physiotherapy with motion exercise of the ankle are necessary. For the first 6 weeks, an ankle-high shoe with a 1 cm wedge under the heel is worn. In case of relevant partial tear repair, the heel raise may be increased. Usually, return to sports is not before 3 months postoperative since tendon healing takes this time to remodel the tendon fibers. During the restructuring process, the tendon is stiffer, and symptoms while doing the first steps in the morning or after sitting are common. Sometimes, this also occurs in combination with a bone bruise of the calcaneus. Medication to support the tendon healing with collagen hydrolysate, glucosamine, and chondroitin sulfate and bone healing such as calcium and vitamin D3 can be of benefit.

9.5 Pearls Tips and Pitfalls

- If the fiber direction for the tendon-splitting incision is difficult to recognize, the dull side of the blade should be used so that the fibers direct the way of the blade.
- While resecting any calcanear spur, it is very important to shape the medial and lateral edges without forgetting any bony formation especially no intratendinous ossification.
- To prevent development of granuloma, bone wax should be applied with only a thin layer.
- For a better tension distribution of the suture, a consecutive suture is recommended.

Endoscopic Technique for Noncalcified Tendinopathy

10

K.T.M. Opdam, J.I. Wiegerinck,
and C. Niek van Dijk

10.1 Indication and Diagnosis

Retrocalcaneal bursitis is an inflammation of the bursa located in the retrocalcaneal recess between the anterior aspect of the Achilles tendon and the posterosuperior part of the calcaneus. The inflammation is caused by repetitive impingement between the ventral side of the Achilles tendon and the posterosuperior calcaneal prominence. Patients present themselves with a typical pain when starting to walk after a period of rest. It can occur bilaterally, mainly in women and often at the end of the second or third decade. A distinction must be made between retrocalcaneal bursitis, superficial calcaneal bursitis, and insertional and midportion Achilles tendinopathy. This distinction can be made by acquiring a detailed medical history and physical examination (Figs. 10.1 and 10.2).

In case of retrocalcaneal bursitis, a swelling is seen, at the level of the posterosuperior calcaneal prominence, on both sides of the Achilles tendon [4]. Superficial calcaneal bursitis is visible as a posterolateral swelling and is locally painful on palpation. Insertional Achilles tendinopathy often coexists with retrocalcaneal bursitis and is painful on palpation at the insertion of the calcaneus. Midportion Achilles tendinopathy gives complaints more proximal than the other pathologies.

The first step in diagnostic imaging is conventional radiographs. The pre-Achilles fat pad, also known as the Kager fat pad, is assessed on a lateral weight-bearing radiograph and is a triangular-shaped radiolucent area with sharp, gently curving borders [1]. In the posteroinferior corner of the pad, the retrocalcaneal bursa is situated. In case of bursitis, the bursa obliterates the normally sharply outlined radiolucent retrocalcaneal recess. If uncertainty about the diagnosis remains, additional investigation should be performed in the form of an ultrasound or MRI.

In case conservative treatment consisting of adaption of the shoe, insoles, nonsteroidal inflammatory drugs, and stretching the gastrocnemius-soleus complex fails, there is a need for other options. When the retrocalcaneal bursitis is chronic, corticosteroids can be injected. However, when conservative treatment fails, surgery must be considered. A well-established treatment option is endoscopic calcaneoplasty, because this offers the advantages of minimally invasive surgery compared with open surgical approaches, like low morbidity, short duration of surgery and short in hospital stay, smaller scars, shorter rehabilitation time, and a quicker resumption of sport [2, 5].

K.T.M. Opdam • J.I. Wiegerinck • C.N. van Dijk (✉)
Academic Medical Center, Department of Orthopedic Surgery, Meibergdreef 9, 1105 AZ Amsterdam, The Netherlands
e-mail: k.t.opdam@amc.uva.nl; j.i.wiegerinck@amc.uva.nl; c.n.vandijk@amc.uva.nl

© ESSKA 2017
H. Thermann et al. (eds.), *The Achilles Tendon*, DOI 10.1007/978-3-662-54074-9_10

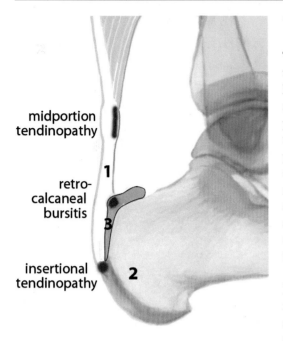

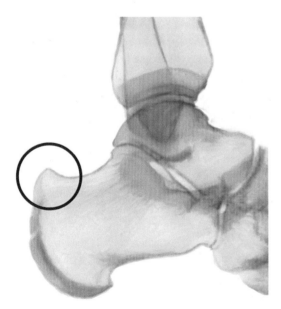

Fig. 10.1 Drawing of the typical location of tenderness. (1 = Achilles tendon, 2 = calcaneus, 3 = retrocalcaneal bursa)

10.2   Operative Setup

The procedure is performed as outpatient surgery under general anesthesia or epidural anesthesia. Preoperatively, the affected side is marked to avoid surgery on the wrong side. The patient is placed in a prone position with the feet just over the edge of the operating table, and a small support is placed under the lower leg, making it possible to move the ankle freely. The anatomical structures are marked; these include the medial and lateral border of the Achilles tendon and the calcaneus. After exsanguination a tourniquet is applied around the affected upper leg and inflated to 300 mmHg.

For irrigation normal saline is used; however, Ringer's solution is also possible. Gravity inflow is adequate for irrigation. When needed a pressure bag is inflated up to 100 mmHg. A 4.0 mm arthroscope with an inclination angle of 30° is routinely used. Furthermore, a probe and 5.5 mm bonecutter shaver are needed.

Fig. 10.2 Lateral view of the ankle shows bone formation at the level of the posterosuperior border of the calcaneus

10.3 Surgical Technique

Two portals are used to perform endoscopic calcaneoplasty. It can be difficult to palpate the superior part of the calcaneus due to swelling, causing you to place the portals to proximal and making the calcaneus difficult to access. Van Dijk et al. standardized the portals for hindfoot endoscopy [3]. The distal tip of the fibula is used as a landmark for placement of the portals, just posteromedial and posterolateral to the Achilles tendon. With the ankle in a plantigrade position, a line is drawn parallel to the foot sole through the tip of the lateral malleolus toward the Achilles tendon. For endoscopic calcaneoplasty the portals are placed 15–20 mm below this line (Fig. 10.3).

First, the lateral portal is made by making a vertical stab incision through the skin at the level of the superior aspect of the calcaneus, just lateral to the Achilles tendon. After that the retrocalcaneal space is penetrated by a blunt trocar. A 4.5 mm 30° arthroscopic shaft is introduced to inspect the retrocalcaneal bursa. The medial portal is made under direct vision by introducing a spinal needle at the same level as the lateral portal. The second portal is made just medial to the Achilles tendon at the level of the superior aspect of the calcaneus. A vertical stab incision is made and the retrocalcaneal bursa is entered with a mosquito forceps. Subsequently, a 5.5 mm bonecutter shaver is introduced, always facing the bone to prevent iatrogenic damage to the Achilles tendon. The inflamed retrocalcaneal bursa is removed, making it possible to inspect the superior surface of the calcaneus. During the procedure the foot can be brought into full dorsiflexion to assess impingement between the Achilles tendon and the calcaneus. Thereafter, the foot is brought into full plantar flexion, and the calcaneal posterosuperior bone rim is easily removed with the bonecutter. Interchangeable use of the portals is possible for the arthroscope and the bonecutter to remove all the bone prominence. It is important to remove the bone sufficiently at the posteromedial and posterolateral corner and to round off the edges. To round off the edges, the bonecutter shaver is moved beyond the posterior edge onto the lateral medial wall of the calcaneus. To visualize the insertion of the Achilles tendon, the foot is placed in full plantar flexion. The bonecutter shaver can be placed just on the insertion of the Achilles tendon against the calcaneus to smoothen this part of the calcaneus. At the end of the procedure, ensure that sufficient bone is removed by switching portals for inspection (for the surgical steps, see Fig. 10.4).

The skin incisions are sutured with 3.0 Ethilon, to prevent sinus formation, and injected with 10 ml of a 0.5% bupivacaine/morphine solution. Afterward, a sterile compressive dressing is applied.

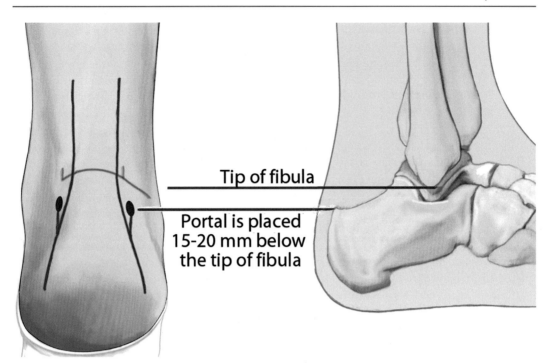

Fig. 10.3 For endoscopic calcaneoplasty, the portals are placed 15–20 mm below the line of the standard two-portal hindfoot technique

Fig. 10.4 (**a**) Lateral view (*left*) shows posterosuperior calcaneal prominence. The *red line* illustrates the level of resection we are aiming at. Drawing of endoscopic view (*right*) showing the posterolateral calcaneal prominence(*), the Achilles tendon (AT), and the insertion of the Achilles tendon onto the calcaneus(**). (**b**) Partial removal of the bone on the lateral side of the calcaneus. (**c**) The shaver is seen at the top of the prominence, placed in the medial portal to further resect the bone. (**d**) Postoperative X-ray (*left*). Endoscopic view of the final situation (*right*) showing the posterolateral calcaneal prominence(*), the Achilles tendon (AT), and the insertion of the Achilles tendon onto the calcaneus(**)

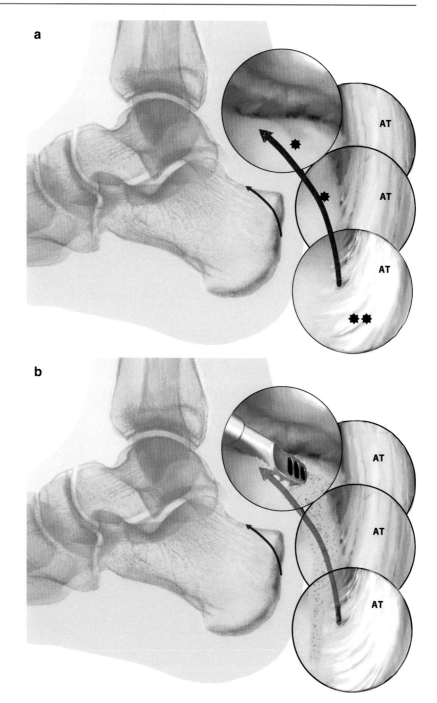

Fig. 10.4 (continued)

10.4   Postoperative Care

Postoperatively, the patient is instructed to elevate the foot when not walking and is allowed weight bearing as tolerated. After 3 days the compressive dressing is removed after which the patient is allowed to shower. From day one, active range of motion exercises are advised for at least three times for 2 min a day. When tolerated normal shoe wear is allowed and the sutures are removed after 2 weeks. A conventional lateral radiograph can be made to ascertain sufficient bone removal. No further outpatient clinic contact is necessary. If there is a limited range of motion, referral to a physiotherapist is advised. Running is allowed from 4 weeks post-op and sport resumption at 6–8 weeks.

10.5   Pearls Tips and Pitfalls

- Throughout the procedure, the Achilles tendon is protected by keeping the closed end of the bonecutter toward the tendon.

- Use two portals interchangeably to ensure that sufficient bone is removed.
- The most frequent cause of remaining complaints after surgery is insufficient resection of the bone. Use intraoperative image intensifier when in doubt.

References

1. Goodman LR, Shanser JD. The pre-Achilles fat pad: an aid to early diagnosis of local or systemic disease. Skeletal Radiol. 1997;2:81–6.
2. Scholten PE, van Dijk CN. Endoscopic calcaneoplasty. Foot Ankle Clin. 2006;11(2):439–46, viii. doi:10.1016/j.fcl.2006.02.004.
3. van Dijk CN, Scholten PE, Krips R. A 2-portal endoscopic approach for diagnosis and treatment of posterior ankle pathology. Arthroscopy. 2000;16(8):871–6. doi:10.1053/jars.2000.19430.
4. van Dijk CN, van Sterkenburg MN, Wiegerinck JI, Karlsson J, Maffulli N. Terminology for Achilles tendon related disorders. Knee Surg Sports Traumatol Arthrosc. 2011;19(5):835–41. doi:10.1007/s00167-010-1374-z.
5. Wiegerinck JI, Kok AC, van Dijk CN. Surgical treatment of chronic retrocalcaneal bursitis. Arthroscopy. 2012;28(2):283–93. doi:10.1016/j.arthro.2011.09.019.

Paul G. Talusan and Lew C. Schon

11.1 Indication and Diagnosis

Patients with insertional Achilles tendinopathy have pain at the bone-tendon interface, limited dorsiflexion, pain with active plantar flexion, pain with passive dorsiflexion, and prominence of the bone-tendon junction. Patients may also have retrocalcaneal bursitis, and in severe cases, the Achilles tendon proximal to the junction may have palpable thickening, warmth, and tenderness.

Radiographs typically demonstrate a Haglund's deformity (prominence of the posterior superior calcaneal tuberosity), intratendinous calcifications, and occasionally an enthesophyte within the tendon.

MRI usually reveals thickening, degenerative tears, and fibrosis. There is juxtatendinous superficial and retrocalcaneal edema. Enlargement of the retrocalcaneal bursa is noted. At the tendon junction, there can be bony and tendon edema. In more severe cases, more proximal tendon changes are noted.

Surgical intervention is indicated when a patient continues to have symptoms following 3–6 months of nonoperative treatment consisting of Achilles stretching, eccentric Achilles strengthening, solid ankle-foot orthoses (off-the-shelf boot braces), heel lifts, and physical therapy.

In most cases, if less than 50% of the tendon remains after debridement, the Achilles tendon can be debrided and reattached without necessitating augmentation. If more than 50% of the tendon is debrided or if there is more proximal involvement of the tendon, then we typically augment with an FDL or FHL transfer. The patient should be consented for this potential augmentation preoperatively. If inadequate length of the Achilles tendon remains after debridement, we counsel the patient about a potential V-Y lengthening or Strayer procedure which necessitates a longer incision.

Contraindications to this elective procedure are patients with active infection, open local ulcerations, heavy smokers, vascular insufficiency, uncontrolled diabetes, and patients with limited functional demands.

P.G. Talusan, MD
Department of Orthopaedic Surgery,
University of Michigan, Ann Arbor, MI, USA
e-mail: ptalusan@med.umich.edu

L.C. Schon, MD (✉)
Department of Orthopaedic Surgery,
MedStar Union Memorial Hospital,
Baltimore, MD, USA
e-mail: lewschon1@gmail.com

11.2 Operative Setup

In addition to the standard instruments used in typical foot and ankle surgery, a mini C-arm, microsagittal saw, chisels, bone rasp, and suture anchors should be available. We perform the surgery in the prone position, but if the patient is overweight or has a difficult airway, sleep apnea,

© ESSKA 2017
H. Thermann et al. (eds.), *The Achilles Tendon*, DOI 10.1007/978-3-662-54074-9_11

or other medical risks, supine "sloppy" lateral with the affected foot down is recommended.

Standard prone positioning or supine "sloppy" lateral with the affected foot down is recommended as mentioned above with generous padding of bony prominences. Ensure that appropriate lateral imaging of the heel can be obtained with the mini C-arm prior to draping; this can be accomplished with knee flexion (prone position) or with abduction (supine position) of the operative limb. Skin preparation is with a chlorhexidine solution to the level of the knee, and a sterile towel and extremity drape are then placed.

We do not typically use a tourniquet. If a tourniquet is used, it should be applied while the patient is supine on the stretcher prior to flipping onto the operating room table because placing a tourniquet on a prone patient is difficult. It should be placed on the thigh to avoid any tethering of the gastrocnemius which would inhibit appropriate tensioning of the Achilles tendon.

We prefer sedation with an ankle block but a general anesthetic can also be used. We perform an ankle block of the superficial peroneal, deep peroneal, saphenous, sural, and tibial nerves approximately 5 cm proximal to the ankle joint using a 40 mL mixture consisting of 20 mL of 1% lidocaine and 20 mL of 0.25% bupivacaine without epinephrine. An additional incisional infiltration can be critical to a successful block.

Antibiotic prophylaxis with a third-generation cephalosporin is instilled 20 min prior to incision. A sequential compression device is placed on the contralateral leg for thrombosis prophylaxis.

11.3   Surgical Technique

A central splitting 8 cm incision that begins 2 cm proximal to the Achilles insertion is made and deepened through the tendon to the bone. The skin flap should be thick and includes skin, fat, and paratenon (Fig. 11.1).

The bone is resected using a microsagittal saw and a chisel. Care is taken to keep the bone cut about 20–30 degrees off the line of the tendon. It is possible to inadvertently progress at too steep of an angle and violate the subtalar joint. The medial and lateral sides of the calcaneus may require a chamfer cut to bevel the edge of the calcaneus (Fig. 11.2).

One 5.0 mm suture anchor with four strands of #2 suture is placed centrally in the calcaneus. Occasionally two anchors are used and one is placed medially and one laterally. These anchors are at the insertion site of the Achilles (Fig. 11.3).

A running Krakow-style suture is passed proximally and distally on each side of the tendon. One strand runs up and down the medial side and one strand up and down the lateral side. Then use the other strand to pull the tendon to the anchor and tie it. Make sure to bury the knot (Figs. 11.4 and 11.5).

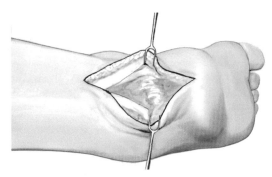

Fig. 11.1 A central splitting 8 cm incision that begins 2 cm proximal to the Achilles insertion is made and deepened through the tendon to the bone

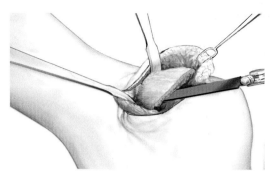

Fig. 11.2 Resect the Haglund's deformity using a micro-sagittal saw. Avoid violating the subtalar joint. The medial and lateral sides of the calcaneus may require a chamfer cut to bevel the edge of the calcaneus

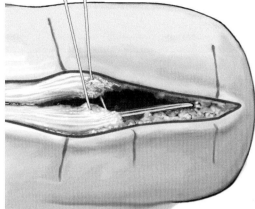

Fig. 11.4 A running Krakow-style suture is passed proxi-mally and distally on each side of the tendon

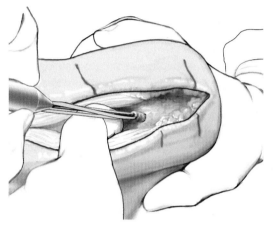

Fig. 11.3 A 5.0 mm corkscrew anchor with four strands of #2 suture is placed centrally. Occasionally two anchors are used and one is placed medially and one laterally

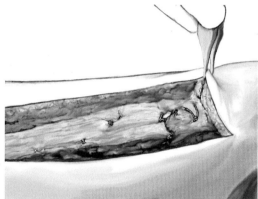

Fig. 11.5 One strand runs up and down the medial side and one strand up and down the lateral side. Then use the other strand to pull the tendon to the anchor and tie it

11.4 Postoperative Care

We close the incision with subcuticular inter-rupted 2-0 and 4-0 Vicryl, running 4-0 Monocryl suture, and Steri-Strips. A well-padded plaster posterior U splint is applied with the ankle in 20 degrees of plantar flexion.

Ten to fourteen days after surgery, the splint is removed, and the patient is placed into a remov-able boot with a heel wedge to achieve 20 degrees of plantar flexion. The boot is worn when the patient is ambulating with crutches or using a rolling knee scooter. The brace is typically removed for sleeping, showering, and resting to allow for gentle range of motion from 10 to 50 degrees of ankle plantar flexion, active inversion and eversion, and toe flexion and extension.

At 6 weeks postoperatively, the heel wedge is removed, and range of motion increases from neutral to 50 degrees of plantar flexion. Patients are typically non-weightbearing for the first 6 weeks after surgery, and a postoperative weight-bearing protocol is initiated. If only the central aspect of the tendon was detached and the lateral and medial bands of the tendon remain, patients may begin weightbearing at 10 days in the boot.

We typically use 325 mg aspirin daily for deep vein thrombosis prophylaxis unless the patient has a family history or past medical history of thrombotic events. In cases with high risk of deep vein thrombosis, we prescribe low molecular weight heparin daily for 6 weeks.

11.5 Pearls, Tips, and Pitfalls

- Be sure to debride all degenerated tendon. Any remaining tendinopathy may be a source of pain generation and recurrence of symptoms.
- In addition to resecting the Haglund's defor-mity, the medial and lateral edges of the calca-neus may need to be filed down with a rasp to smooth any remaining rough edges.
- There are often enthesophytes on the posterior surface of the tuberosity which should be resected at the time of surgery. Intraoperative fluoroscopy can be used to ensure total resec-tion of this pathologic structure.
- Proper tensioning of the Achilles tendon is critical, and evaluation of the contralateral side is helpful in determining proper tension.

Part IV

Delayed Reconstruction of Achilles Tendon Rupture

Open Reconstruction with Gastrocnemius V-Y Advancement

12

Andrew R. Hsu, Bruce E. Cohen, and Robert B. Anderson

12.1 Indication and Diagnosis

Achilles pain and dysfunction often result from neglected Achilles ruptures more than 6 weeks old. Chronic ruptures can lead to functional loss due to retraction with tendon fibrosis and atrophy, lengthening of the gastrocnemius-soleus complex, and decreased push-off strength. Pain is typically found within the mid-substance of the tendon or at its insertion with associated ankle and calf weakness. Chronic ruptures commonly occur in patients in the fourth to fifth decades of life and may result from neglected acute partial ruptures, progressive microtears and scarring, and/or drug-induced tendon breakdown (i.e., fluoroquinolones).

During physical exam patients with chronic ruptures often ambulate with a limp and have difficulty standing on the affected extremity and performing a single-limb heel rise. There is often a nodularity, fullness, crepitance, and/or palpable gap within the tendon indicating the location of a previous partial or complete rupture. It is important to evaluate skin quality, tendon strength, and

tendon continuity (Thompson test) during clinical exam. Resting Achilles tension should be compared to the contralateral side along with the degree of calf atrophy. Posterior heel pain can also be present as a result of associated Haglund deformity, retrocalcaneal bursitis, insertional Achilles tendinitis, or a combination of the above.

Standard lateral radiographs of the affected extremity may show a Haglund deformity, calcifications within the tendon, and/or a calcaneal avulsion injury. Calcific deposits within the Achilles tendon often require open debridement (Fig. 12.1). Ultrasound can be used to identify nodules, cysts, and large tendon defects. MRI can help assess for tendinosis and bursitis in the area of rupture along with the size of the defect and the condition of the proximal and distal extents of tendon. Prior to Achilles reconstruction, chronic Achilles ruptures can be treated non-operatively with heel lifts (2–3 cm) and orthotics, ankle-foot orthosis (AFO) bracing, nonsteroidal anti-inflammatory drugs (NSAIDs), standard physical therapy with eccentric exercises, modalities such as phonophoresis and/or iontophoresis, or immobilization in a cast or tall controlled ankle motion (CAM) boot. Long-term bracing with an AFO can be used in older, heavier, low-demand patients with significant comorbidities such as diabetes and rheumatoid arthritis. In general, we have found that non-operative treatment for chronic Achilles ruptures other than bracing and symptomatic care does not provide good long-term clinical and functional outcomes.

A.R. Hsu, MD
University of California-Irvine Department of Orthopaedic Surgery, Orange, CA 92868, USA
e-mail: hsuar@uci.edu

B.E. Cohen, MD • R.B. Anderson, MD (✉)
Foot & Ankle Institute, OrthoCarolina, Charlotte, NC 28207, USA
e-mail: bruce.cohen@orthocarolina.com; robert.anderson@orthocarolina.com

© ESSKA 2017
H. Thermann et al. (eds.), *The Achilles Tendon*, DOI 10.1007/978-3-662-54074-9_12

There are some literature and anecdotal reports advocating for the use of topical NSAIDs and glyceryl trinitrate, platelet-rich plasma injections, and extracorporeal shockwave therapy. We do not routinely employ these modalities due to logistical and cost reasons as well as the lack of supporting scientific evidence.

Open Achilles reconstruction is recommended in patients who remain symptomatic despite thorough use of non-operative treatments. Additional indications include chronic pain refractory to bracing and loss of plantar flexion strength negatively affecting quality of life. We have found that most healthy, active patients with chronic Achilles ruptures will typically re-present to clinic after 3–6 months of non-operative treatment with persistent pain and ankle weakness. We have also found that the majority of athletes do poorly with non-operative intervention and are unable to return to baseline activities.

Surgical management is determined by the size of the Achilles defect and the quality of the gastrocnemius-soleus muscle complex. We have found that defects 1–2 cm in size can be spanned with a traditional direct repair using locked Krackow sutures and overlying reinforcement sutures. A gastrocnemius fascial lengthening can be added to increase excursion length as needed. For defects 2–5 cm in length, we recommend gastrocnemius V-Y fascial advancement to mobilize the musculotendinous unit and decrease the defect size.

Surgical intervention is generally contraindicated in patients with active infection, uncontrolled diabetes, peripheral neuropathy, severe peripheral vascular disease, and/or medical comorbidities that significantly increase the risks of surgery. The potential benefits of increased tendon strength and decreased chance of re-rupture with surgical

intervention must be carefully weighed against the risk of wound complications and infection. All potential risks, benefits, and alternatives of surgical treatment should be discussed in full with patients along with the necessary rehabilitation protocol.

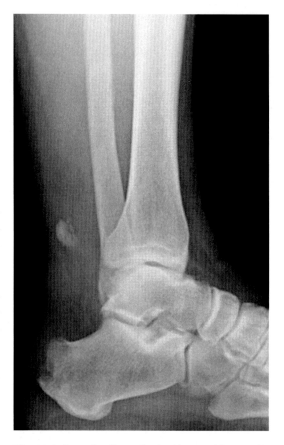

Fig. 12.1 Lateral radiograph of a 43-year-old man with neglected right Achilles tendon rupture. Patient had a baseline Haglund deformity and insertional Achilles tendinitis and sustained an avulsion fracture off the insertion of the Achilles tendon. On exam and X-rays 3 months after his avulsion injury, he was found to have large calcific deposits within the tendon requiring open debridement and tendon reconstruction

12.2 Operative Setup

Patients are anesthetized using general anesthesia in combination with popliteal and saphenous nerve blocks. While supine, a tourniquet is placed high on the operative leg before flipping the patient prone.

Chest and knee pads are placed on the operating room table followed by careful flipping of the patient into the prone position with the feet located at the end of the bed. Bilateral upper extremities are positioned at right angles at the level of the shoulders under pads to reduce the incidence of brachial plexus stretch and injury. All prominences are checked to ensure that they are properly padded. Pillows are placed underneath the bilateral tibias to reduce stretch on the sciatic nerve.

The operative extremity is then prepped from the foot to the popliteal crease using 2% chlorhexidine gluconate in combination with 70% isopropyl alcohol (ChloraPrep®, CareFusion, San Diego, CA).

12.3 Surgical Technique

The operative extremity is exsanguinated using an Esmarch bandage and the tourniquet inflated. Separate midline incisions are marked proximally and distally for the gastrocnemius V-Y advancement and Achilles reconstruction, respectively (Fig. 12.2). The skin is incised followed by careful dissection and incision of the paratenon for later repair. A "no-touch" technique is employed in which the skin and superficial tissues are not grasped with pickups to reduce the incidence of soft tissue damage.

The Achilles is evaluated for the presence of fibrotic tissue and tendinosis, and all unhealthy tissue and calcifications are sharply excised back to healthy-appearing striated tendon (Fig. 12.3). There is often a large mid-substance gap after debridement that should be measured in order to evaluate the need for a gastrocnemius advancement. We have found that a gastrocnemius advancement can reliably and reproducibly compensate for up to a 4–5 cm defect in the Achilles tendon (Fig. 12.3). The proximal incision is then made, and the sural nerve must be identified and carefully dissected out of the way as it is often located in the operative field. A V-shaped incision is marked on the proximal gastrocnemius fascia with the apex of the V pointing proximally and with the sural nerve gently moved to the side (Fig. 12.4). The length of each arm of the V-shaped incision should be 1.5 times the size of the defect. It is important that the V be centered in the gastrocnemius fascia after adjustment for rotation of the leg due to patient positioning.

A Kocher or Allis clamp is placed on the proximal Achilles stump through the distal incision in order to place the gastrocnemius fascia under tension to allow for easier incision. After incising the V in the gastrocnemius, the fascia is separated from the underlying soleus bluntly with a finger or sharply with Metzenbaum scissors in order to ensure that there are no more remaining raphe or remaining adhesions. It is critical to free-up any potential adhesions in order to maximize tendon excursion and allow for end-to-end apposition of the Achilles tendon stumps (Fig. 12.5). After Achilles tendon apposition is achieved, the gastrocnemius proximal Y limb is closed while applying gentle tension using interrupted 2-0 Vicryl sutures (Ethicon, Somerville, NJ) followed by closure of the medial and lateral limbs.

The Achilles tendon stumps are then sharply debrided of any frayed edges that may block repair. The stumps are repaired end to end with the ankle plantar-flexed position using #2 FiberWire (Arthrex, Naples, FL) with locking Krackow sutures so that two knots are buried within the rupture site. Krackow sutures on one side are tied securely while holding tension on the opposite side in order to prevent suture from pulling through the tendon. The repair is then supplemented with buried 0 Vicryl sutures and an epitendinous 2-0 Vicryl suture to smooth down the edges of the repair site, increase strength, and tubularize the tendon (Fig. 12.6). The operative extremity is flexed 90° at the knee, and the resting tension of the Achilles repair is checked along with a Thompson test to ensure tendon continuity and excursion.

The wound is thoroughly irrigated, and subcutaneous tissues are closed with buried interrupted 3-0 Monocryl sutures (Ethicon, Somerville, NJ) followed by interrupted 3-0 nylon sutures for skin closure (Fig. 12.2). A non-adherent soft dressing is applied followed by placement of a non-weight-bearing short leg splint with the ankle in its resting plantar-flexed position.

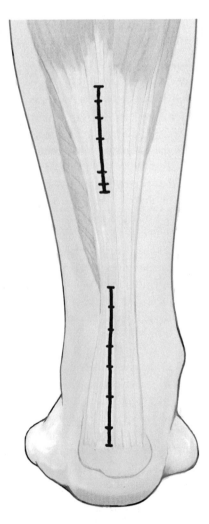

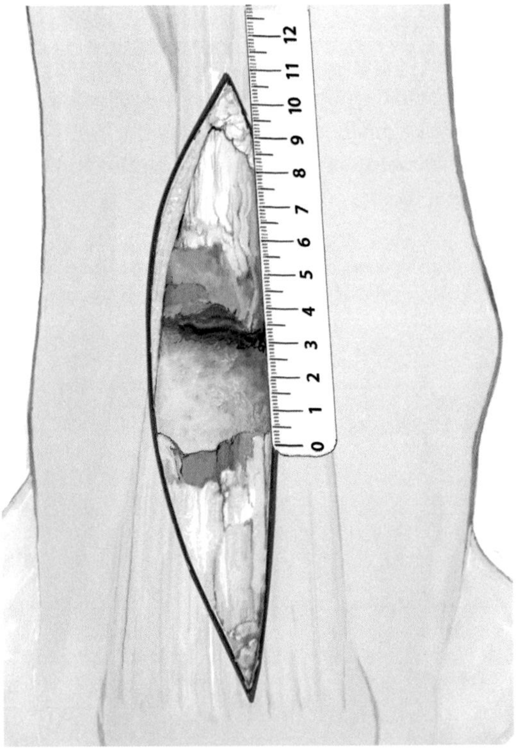

Fig. 12.3 Remaining 4 cm mid-substance gap in Achilles after debridement and excision of fibrotic tissue, abnormal tendon, and calcific deposits

Fig. 12.2 Planned midline proximal and distal incisions for gastrocnemius V-Y advancement and Achilles reconstruction, respectively, with patient in the prone position

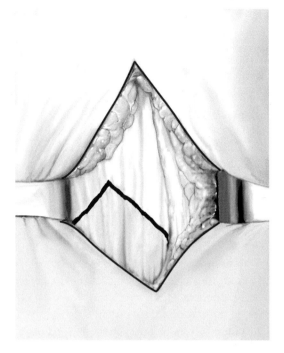

Fig. 12.4 Planned V-shaped gastrocnemius fascia incision for V-Y advancement with dissection and mobilization of sural nerve (right side of wound)

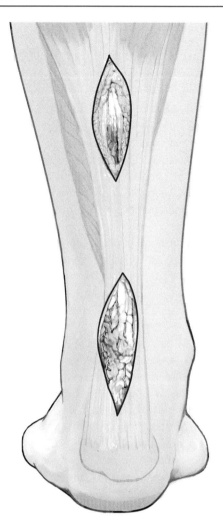

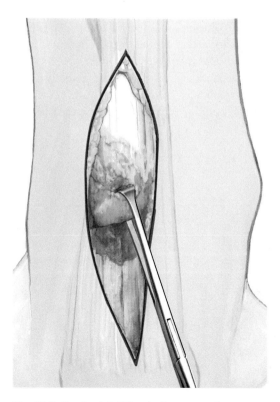

Fig. 12.6 V-Y gastrocnemius advancement closed with 2-0 Vicryl sutures. Achilles repaired end to end with ankle in plantar-flexed position using #2 FiberWire with locking Krackow sutures in the proximal and distal tendon stumps. Achilles repair supplemented with buried 0 Vicryl sutures along with an epitendinous 2-0 Vicryl suture

Fig. 12.5 Proximal Achilles tendon stump advancement of 4 cm after V-Y advancement allowing direct repair

12.4 Postoperative Care

Functional outcome after Achilles reconstruction is strongly correlated with patient compliance, postoperative rehabilitation, and physical therapy. Patients are immobilized non-weight bearing in a short leg splint placed in plantar flexion for 2 weeks after surgery to allow for initial wound healing. If the wound is healed at 2 weeks, sutures are removed, and patients are placed in a tall CAM boot with continued non-weight bearing and initiation of gentle active ankle range of motion for 2 weeks. If the wound is not fully healed, if patients have questionable compliance, or if the surgical repair was noted to be tenuous at the time of surgery, patients are kept non-weight bearing in a short leg cast for an additional 2 weeks. At 4 weeks after surgery, all patients are transitioned to partial weight bearing (50%) in a tall CAM boot with peel-away heel lifts (2 cm) that can be sequentially removed to reduce the amount of plantar flexion every 3 days.

The goal is to have patients fully weight bearing without any heel lifts at 6 weeks post-op. The tall CAM boot is maintained until 8–10 weeks post-op at which time patients are weaned out of the boot into a normal accommodative shoe. From 8–12 weeks patients participate in physical therapy working on stretching, strengthening, and range of motion exercises to the operative extremity. Therapy is continued from weeks 12–16 to increase muscle strength and activity level while avoiding running or other impact exercises. At 16 weeks after surgery, patients are released to perform all activities as tolerated including impact athletics. In our experiences, we have found that the general patient population requires 8–12 months to fully recover to baseline activities after open Achilles reconstruction. We have also found that athletes require 6–8 months to return to play depending on the sport and position played.

12.5 Pearls, Tips, and Pitfalls

- A gastrocnemius V-Y advancement can be used to manage chronic Achilles defects 2–5 cm in length.
- A "no-touch" technique should be used to reduce soft tissue injury during dissection.
- It is important to sharply excise all fibrosis and tendinosis back to healthy tissue prior to repair.
- The V-shaped incision needs to be centered in the fascia, and each arm should be 1.5 times the size of the defect.
- All adhesions should be freed to maximize tendon excursion and reduce tension on the end-to-end repair.
- Krackow sutures should be combined with epitendinous sutures to smooth down the edges of the repair site and increase strength.

Free/Turndown Gastrocnemius Flap Augmentation

13

Katarina Nilsson-Helander, Leif Swärd,
Michael R. Carmont, Nicklas Olsson,
and Jon Karlsson

13.1 Indication and Diagnosis

Surgical treatment is recommended for a chronic Achilles tendon rupture, as well as a re-rupture. Chronic Achilles tendon ruptures are referred to those more than 4 weeks after initial injury. An end-to-end repair is considered insufficient for tendons with a chronic injury or re-rupture and reinforcement is recommended. Fascial reinforcement has not been shown to improve outcome for acute ruptures.

Several techniques have been described in the literature to augment end-to-end repairs and bridge gaping between the tendon ends in non-apposed reconstructions. Whilst repairs augmented with free tendon transfer are very strong, they are also bulky and this may prevent closure of the overlying fascia cruris.

The fascia of the calf, the fascia cruris, is closely linked to the underling paratenon and from which the Achilles tendon receives its blood supply. In addition the fascia provides stability to the overlying skin and optimizes skin perfusion by maintaining arteriole tension and as a consequence patency. Following chronic Achilles rupture, the fascia and paratenon thicken and adapt to a deficient non-apposed rupture site. It may not be subsequently possible to close the fascia over a bulky reconstruction with normal fascial tension. If the fascia is closed with tension potentially reducing the blood supply to the underlying reconstruction and the overlying skin increasing the chance of wound breakdown.

A fascial graft from the gastrocnemius aponeurosis provides a strong, easily accessible, low bulk graft to augment end-to-end repairs in cases of nonunion and re-rupture. Small gaps can be bridged using a free gastrocnemius patch [1], whereas larger defects can be reconstructed using a turndown flap, which may be reversed [2]. There is no morbidity or weakness from tendon transfer.

The use of a small free flap permits a smaller incision over the repair site, possibly reducing the tendency to wound breakdown. Although the turndown flap requires a much longer incision, in our hands, the low bulk of this graft means that wound breakdown is a rare occurrence [1].

K. Nilsson-Helander • L. Swärd • N. Olsson
J. Karlsson (✉)
The Department of Orthopaedic Surgery,
Sahlgrenska Academy, University of Gothenburg,
Gothenburg, Sweden

Department of Orthopaedic, Kungsbacka Hospital,
Kungsbacka, Sweden
e-mail: Ina.nilsson@telia.com; Leif.sward@me.com;
nicklas.olsson@gu.se; Jon.Karlsson@telia.com

M.R. Carmont
The Department of Orthopaedic Surgery,
Princess Royal Hospital, Shrewsbury, UK

Telford Hospital NHS Trust, Shropshire, UK
e-mail: mcarmont@hotmail.com

© ESSKA 2017
H. Thermann et al. (eds.), *The Achilles Tendon*, DOI 10.1007/978-3-662-54074-9_13

13.2   Operative Setup

A laminar flow operating theatre is preferable. The patient is positioned prone using a thigh tourniquet applied prior to turning. Two applications of 2% chlorhexidine skin preparation are used up to the tourniquet.

13.3   Surgical Technique

A longitudinal incision 20–25 cm long is used (Fig. 13.1). This is commenced distally medial to the Achilles tendon and extended proximally as required curving towards the midline. Care should be taken to avoid injuring the sural nerve as this structure becomes more midline at the calf.

An end-to-end suture, using a modified Kessler suturing technique with 1-0 PDS, is applied after careful debridement of interposed scar tissue (Fig. 13.2).

The free flap is harvested from the gastrocnemius aponeurosis (Fig. 13.3). The size of the tendon gap decides the length, width and thickness of the free flap. Usually it is sufficient with a width/length of 3–5/3–7 cm. The thickness of the flap depends on the remaining gap after modified Kessler suturing. The free flap is placed over the gap with the deep side downside (Fig. 13.4) against the apposed repair and then secured, using 3-0 PDS (Fig. 13.5).

The wound is carefully closed, aiming at low tension. The fascia cruris and paratenon are then closed using detensioning mattress sutures. In addition detensioning subcutaneous and skin mattress sutures with 3,0 nylon are applied (Fig. 13.6).

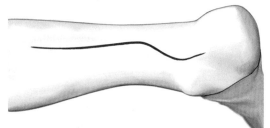

Fig. 13.1 A longitudinal (20–25 cm length), proximal central to a slightly medially curved distal skin incision is used (avoid sural nerve injury)

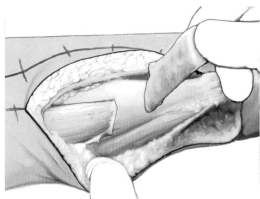

Fig. 13.3 A free gastrocnemius aponeurosis flap is prepared. The size of the tendon gap decides the length, width and thickness of the fee flap. Usually it is sufficient with a width/length of 3–5/3–7 cm. The thickness of the flap depends on the remaining gap after modified Kessler suturing

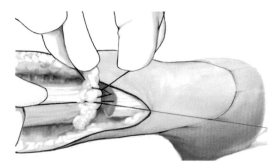

Fig. 13.2 An end-to-end suture, using a modified Kessler suturing technique with 1-0 PDS, is applied after debridement of scar tissue

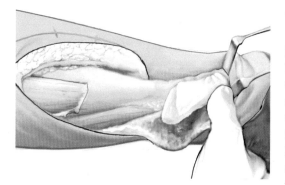

Fig. 13.4 The relatively vascular muscular side of the fascia to be applied against the reconstruction

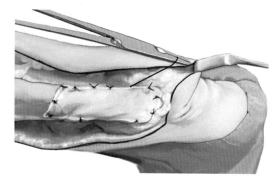

Fig. 13.5 The free flap is then secured, using 3-0 PDS, covering the gap

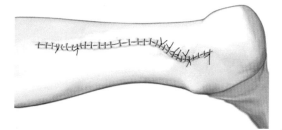

Fig. 13.6 After flap reinforcement, the wound is carefully closed, aiming at low tension

13.4 Post-operative Care

Following surgery, patients were placed into a below knee cast with the foot in equinus for 3 weeks. After this the position of the cast was changed to neutral for a further 3 weeks. At 6 weeks following surgery, the patient commenced free range of motion training using a movable lower leg brace. Full weight bearing was started at 6 weeks. The moveable lower leg brace was removed 8 weeks after surgery.

All patients followed a symptom and function criterion-based rehabilitation protocol supervised by a physiotherapist twice a week. Patients started strength training of the gastrocnemius/soleus complex, initially concentric contraction, and the intensity was successively increased. Patients started with two-legged toe raises where possible depending upon the muscle strength and ROM was increased.

13.5 Pearl Tips and Pitfalls

- Commence the incision distally on the medial side of the Achilles tendon and if required extended proximally by curving towards the midline taking care to avoid the sural nerve.
- When the patch is prepared, it must be appreciated that a demarcated flap will retract after its tension is released and the free flap can appear to "shrink," so it is recommended that a slightly larger flap should be dissected than thought to be required.
- In some case it may be necessary to harvest a flap from the ventral aspect of the gastrocnemius aponeurosis.
- To minimize the potential for adhesion formation, the flap should be positioned so that the sliding external surface is superficial to the repair. This is in similar to the folding/reversal of a turndown flap using the Silfverskiöld technique.

References

1. Nilsson-Helander K, Swärd L, Grävare Silbernagel K, Thomeé R, Eriksson BI, Karlsson J. A new surgical method to treat chronic ruptures and re-ruptures of the Achilles tendon. Knee Surg Sports Traumatol Arthrosc. 2008;16(6):614–20.

2. Silfverskiöld N. Über die subkutane toale Achillesshnenruptur und deren Behandling. Acta Chir Scand. 1941;84:393–413.

Free Hamstring Open Augmentation for Delayed Achilles Tendon Rupture

14

Michael R. Carmont, Karin Grävare Silbernagel, Katarina Nilsson-Helander, and Jon Karlsson

14.1 Indication and Diagnosis

Open reconstruction of the Achilles tendon may be considered to be a relatively simple technique and may be easily performed by surgeons less familiar with more complex Achilles reconstruction. The technique may be used for both chronic rupture greater than 4 weeks following injury and cases of re-rupture.

The open method allows bridging of a gap following debridement of the ruptured tendon ends and/or augmentation of an end-to-end repair. An advantage includes a smaller incision compared with fascial turndown or fascial patch techniques. One disadvantage is the relatively bulky nature of the augmentation. In cases of reconstruction, however, the final construct is usually only slightly bulkier than a primary open repair.

Although no research has been performed on the biomechanical properties of interposed pseudotendon tissue, it is likely to be more flexible, retain and release less energy, and elongate more over time, than interposed free tendon autograft. The resection of pseudotendon tissue allows the true defect in the tendon to be determined.

The use of open reconstruction allows the determination of the mode of failure for re-ruptures initially treated operatively. This is particularly important where minimally invasive or percutaneous initial surgery has been performed. Causes include knot failure, suture cutout and misplacement, additional rupture at a different site, or lengthening due to unknown causes (Fig. 14.1).

M.R. Carmont (✉)
The Department of Orthopaedic Surgery,
Princess Royal Hospital, Shrewsbury, UK

Telford Hospital NHS Trust, Shropshire, UK
e-mail: mcarmont@hotmail.com

K.G. Silbernagel
The Department of Physical Therapy,
University of Delaware, Newark, DE, USA
e-mail: kgs@udel.edu

K. Nilsson-Helander • J. Karlsson
The Department of Orthopaedic Surgery,
Sahlgrenska Academy, University of Gothenburg,
Gothenburg, Sweden
e-mail: Ina.nilsson@telia.com;
Jon.Karlsson@telia.com

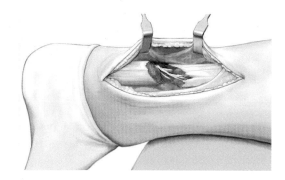

Fig. 14.1 A medial incision revealing the mode of failure of primary repair with suture pullout from the distal stump

© ESSKA 2017
H. Thermann et al. (eds.), *The Achilles Tendon*, DOI 10.1007/978-3-662-54074-9_14

14.2 Operative Setup

A laminar flow operating theater is preferable. The patient is positioned in the recovery position laterally described by Gougoulias [1], with the operated side down. The thigh tourniquet should be applied prior to turning. Care must be taken to ensure that the lower shoulder is flexed to prevent venous compression. The pelvis is tilted and the operated leg, lower leg, is externally rotated. The opposite hip and knee are flexed, and a supportive strap may be applied around the knee to support the pelvis reducing rotational forces on the lumbar spine. Two applications of 2% chlorhexidine skin preparation are used up to the tourniquet.

14.3 Surgical Technique

Based upon operative experience, hamstring harvest may be performed, from the affected side, either with the knee flexed or on the medial aspect of the popliteal fossa [2] (Fig. 14.2).

Surgeons more familiar with hamstring harvest for knee or ankle ligament reconstruction may prefer performing harvest with the knee flexed. Through a longitudinal incision over the pes anserinus, the gracilis tendon can be palpated through the sartorial fascia by rolling beneath the surgeon's fingertip. The fascia is then split in line with the tendon and the tendon harvested according to surgeon's standard technique.

The most familiar method may be to harvest the graft with the patient supine and then reposition the patient. A whip suture is applied to both ends of the graft using either a looped suture or a 45° suture so that tension on the whip suture leads to tendon constriction for easier passage.

With the knee now extended, a medial incision for cosmesis or a midline incision to incorporate a previous surgical scar may be performed. Care must be taken not to undermine the skin edges. Deeper dissection is performed down to the fascia cruris and paratenon. A longitudinal incision

of the paratenon can then be performed to expose the Achilles tendon. The sural nerve lies in the subcutaneous layer and typically crosses the lateral border of the Achilles tendon at 8–10 cm from the insertion on the calcaneum. Knowledge of the course of the nerve and careful dissection minimizes the risk of iatrogenic injury.

The tendon is mobilized proximally and distally, using a blunt dissector, to release adhesions from the fascia cruris and the fascia covering the deep posterior compartment.

The rupture ends are now identified and any pseudotendon excised to tendon end. If end-to-end apposition is impossible due to gaping, a locking suture using No. 1 braided absorbable suture can be placed in the tendon end. The free gracilis graft is then tenodesed to the lateral side of the proximal stump using a Mayo needle (Fig. 14.3).

Transverse coronal tenotomies are then made in the proximal and distal tendon ends of the tendon. The tenotomies should be placed so that there is a 1 cm overlap of tendon and graft. A clip is attached to the tip of the scalpel to facilitate clip passage through the tendon. The clip is then used to grasp the whip suture on either end of the graft (Fig. 14.4).

The tendon is then pulled through the distal stump, and with the ankle held passively in full plantar flexion and tension maintained in the graft, two sutures are applied to the medial and lateral sides of the distal stump. These sutures should maintain the 1 cm overlap.

The graft is then passed transversely through the proximal stump and tenodesed again with four sutures of No. 2 nonabsorbable suture. The ends of the hamstring autograft are now "doubled over," and the Mayo needle is used to tenodese the distal whip suture to the tendon completing the reconstruction with three strands of hamstring bridging the gap between the tendon ends (Fig. 14.5).

The paratenon is then closed using detensioning mattress sutures. In addition detensioning subcutaneous and skin mattress sutures with 3.0 nylon are applied.

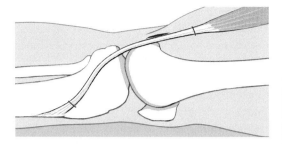

Fig. 14.2 The hamstring tendon is palpable on the medial side of the popliteal fossa with the knee in full extension

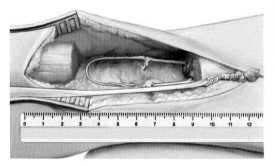

Fig. 14.3 The tendon ends have been resected to stable tendon rather than pseudotendon scar tissue. The whip suture has been used to tenodese the hamstring graft to the proximal tendon stump.

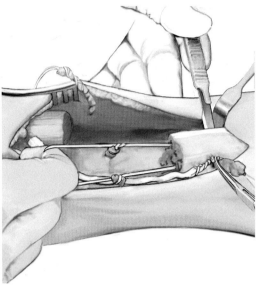

Fig. 14.4 The free graft is passed through coronal plane tenotomies in the distal and sequentially permitting a 1 cm overlap of graft and stump

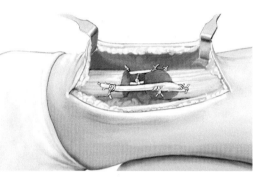

Fig. 14.5 The final reconstruction, end-to-end apposition, was not possible

14.4 Postoperative Care

Postoperatively the patient is placed into a functional brace made from synthetic cast material in equinus. The cast is split and held in place with circumferential Velcro straps. The brace is made preoperatively with the ankle resting in gravity equinus initially and increased manually during the curing of the synthetic cast material.

Elevation during rest is recommended. Toe-touch weight bearing on the metatarsal heads using axillary crutches is permitted for the first 2 weeks. Low molecular weight heparin is administered for this period.

At 2–3 weeks following surgery, sutures are removed and physiotherapy exercises commenced. These consist of active open kinetic chain contraction in plantar flexion, inversion, and eversion, ten times, three times per day. As movement improves resistance, therapeutic band may be used. The posterior shell of the functional brace is removed and weight bearing can be increased. Elbow crutches may be used in preference to axillary crutches encouraging further beneficial loading.

At the 6-week time point, the front shell is discontinued and full weight bearing commenced using a 15 mm heel wedge in the shoe on both feet until the 3-month time point. Formal physiotherapy is commenced with exercises designed to progressively increase the strength and range of motion of the ankle joint. Initially the bilateral standing or seated heel-rises can be initiated to strengthening the calf musculature. The movement should be slow and controlled, and both concentric and eccentric contractions should be performed. The load on the injured leg is progressively increased, and the goal is to be able to achieve a unilateral heel-rise in standing. Other impairments in the lower extremity should also be addressed, and the aim is for the patient to walk without a limp and have normal push-off during gait within the first 3–5 weeks. Local massage can reduce adhesions and swelling. Stretching should be avoided and plyometric exercises should only be permitted at the 3-month time point.

No other time guides are recommended after 3 months, and activities including running and jumping can be introduced when the patient has achieved the ability to perform single-leg heel-rises, can walk without a limb, and has good single-leg balance.

14.5 Pearls, Tips, and Pitfalls

- Hamstring harvest may be difficult. When prone or recovery position, the assistant generally places the knee in flexion rather than holding at 90°. Unfortunately this makes graft harvest more difficult.
- The gracilis tendon is more proximal and cylindrical. This means that gracilis is easier to palpate and recognize beneath the fingertip and harvest. Gracilis also has less accessory bands to the medial gastrocnemius.
- A compressive whip suture, rather than a side suture, helps facilitate graft passage through the tenotomy.
- The free graft elongates with time and rehabilitation. It is recommended to make the reconstruction as tight as possible, in maximal passive ankle plantar flexion.
- One centimeter hamstring overlap with both tendon stump and four sutures significantly improves the strength of the reconstruction.

References

1. Gougoulias N, Dawe EJ, Sakellariou A. The recovery position for posterior of the ankle and hindfoot. Bone Joint J. 2013;95-B:1317–9.
2. Prodromos CC. Posterior mini-incision hamstring harvest. Sports Med Arthrosc. 2010;18(1):12–4.

Minimally Invasive Peroneus Brevis Tendon Transfer

15

Rocco Aicale, Domiziano Tarantino, Francesco Oliva, Michael R. Carmont, and Nicola Maffulli

15.1 Indication and Diagnosis

Transfer of the tendon of peroneus brevis was first proposed for the management of this condition in 1974 [6]. Since then, it has been used successfully in patients with large defects of the Achilles tendon [1]. Miskulin et al. used combined peroneus brevis transfer with augmentation

R. Aicale • D. Tarantino
Department of Musculoskeletal Disorders,
School of Medicine and Surgery, University of Salerno,
Salerno, Italy
e-mail: aicale17@gmail.com;
domiziano22@gmail.com

F. Oliva
Department of Orthopaedic and Traumatology,
University of Rome "Tor Vergata", School of Medicine,
Viale Oxford 81, 00133 Rome, Italy
e-mail: olivafrancesco@hotmail.com

M.R. Carmont
Department of Trauma and Orthopaedic Surgery,
Princess Royal Hospital, Shrewsbury, UK

Telford Hospital NHS Trust, Shropshire, UK
e-mail: mcarmont@hotmail.com

N. Maffulli (✉)
Queen Mary University of London,
Barts and the London School of Medicine and Dentistry,
Centre for Sports and Exercise Medicine,
Mile End Hospital, 275 Bancroft Road,
London E1 4DG, UK

Department of Musculoskeletal Disorders,
School of Medicine and Surgery, University of Salerno,
Salerno, Italy
e-mail: n.maffulli@qmul.ac.uk

of the plantaris tendon for the management of chronic ruptures of the Achilles tendon to supplement function of the Achilles tendon without restoring its anatomy and continuity but reproducing its dynamic function [5]. It must be appreciated that the peroneal muscles provide only 4% of the total work capacity in plantar flexion [3]. Following integration, the peroneus brevis tendon will hypertrophy over time, and its functional incorporation to the Achilles tendon will increase the strength of plantar flexion [7]. Patients may usually return to pre-injury occupation, but not necessarily full function, at mean of 9 weeks (5–16) following surgery. Minimally invasive procedures may be advantageous compared with open techniques, resulting in less wound breakdown, infections and complications [2, 4].

This technique is used for chronic rupture of the Achilles tendon, and the rationale is to supplement the function of the Achilles tendon without restoring its anatomical continuity. Advantages of the described technique include small incisions and the use of tendon transfer supplementation to augment the strength of existing Achilles tendon function. Although eversion strength may be reduced, the weakness of great toe flexion associated with flexor hallucis longus transfer is avoided. Disadvantages include the loss of the muscular function of peroneus brevis. Peroneus brevis contributes 9% of ankle eversion strength, and patients may note ankle instability, with weakened foot pronation until compensated following rehabilitation by peroneus longus and tertius. There is a possibility of avulsion of the transferred tendon, wound breakdown and complex regional pain syndromes together with scar hypersensitivity.

The transfer of the peroneus brevis tendon for the management of chronic ruptures of the Achilles tendon, regardless of the size of the gap, is described. In this technique, the gap in the Achilles tendon is not exposed, and the rationale of the transfer is not to fill a gap but to provide a 'motor', which re-tensions, supplies and augments the function of the gastrocsoleus–Achilles tendon complex [2].

15.2 Operative Setup

Skin preparation and sterile drapes are used. Under general anaesthesia and with the patient prone, a thigh tourniquet is applied, the limb exsanguinated and the tourniquet inflated to 300 mmHg. Intravenous antibiotic prophylaxis, with first-generation cephalosporins, is administered through a dorsal vein of the ipsilateral foot. Postoperative thrombosis prophylaxis is recommended according to patients' risk stratification.

15.3 Surgical Technique

Preoperatively, once the tendon defect has been palpated, the insertion of the Achilles tendon on the calcaneum and the insertion of the peroneus brevis tendon over the base of the fifth metatarsal are identified as landmarks.

A 3 cm longitudinal incision lateral to the midline is used to expose the insertion of the Achilles tendon into the posterolateral corner of the calcaneum, taking care to prevent damage to the sural nerve (Fig. 15.1).

An osteotomy of the posterosuperior corner of the calcaneum is then performed using an oscillating saw (see Sect. 15.3). This prevents impingement of the posterosuperior corner against the Achilles tendon and allows placement of the peroneus brevis tendon closer to the insertion of the Achilles tendon.

A 2.5 cm transverse incision over the base of the fifth metatarsal is then used, and the tendon of peroneus brevis is identified and detached from its insertion into the base of the fifth metatarsal. The distal 3 cm of the peroneus brevis tendon is tubularized with # 1 Vicryl (Ethicon, Edinburgh, United Kingdom) sutures and passed through the proximal incision, beneath the intact bridge of skin (Fig. 15.2).

The proximal portion of the tendon is released from the surrounding tissues and mobilized and the distal edge gently pulled down. The calcaneum is drilled from dorsal to plantar with a Beath pin (Arthrex Inc., Naples, Florida) at an angle of about 45° to the plantar surface of the heel. A cannulated headed reamer of the appropriate diameter is used to drill a tunnel in the calcaneum, through which the peroneus brevis tendon was passed (Fig. 15.3). The transfer is tensioned with the ankle held in maximum equinus. A guide wire is then introduced to place a 7 mm × 20 mm or a 7 mm × 25 mm metallic or bioabsorbable interference screw to secure the tendon of the peroneus brevis to the calcaneum.

The tendon of peroneus brevis is then tenodesed to the distal stump of the Achilles tendon with 2.0 Vicryl sutures (Ethicon).

After irrigation with normal saline, the incisions are closed and Steri-Strips (3M Health Care, St. Paul, Minnesota) applied. A below-knee weight-bearing synthetic cast is applied with the ankle in maximal plantar flexion, leaving the metatarsal heads free.

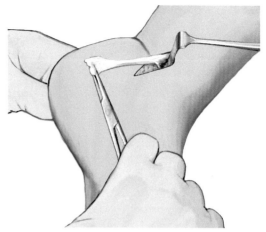

Fig. 15.2 The peroneus brevis tendon is mobilized and pulled distally after accurate removal of peritendinous adhesions

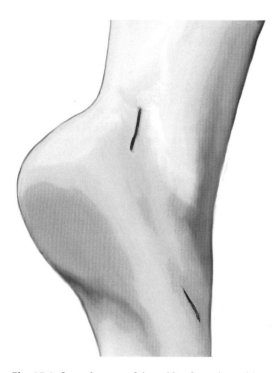

Fig. 15.1 Lateral aspect of the ankle of a patient with a chronic tear of the Achilles tendon. The patient is prone. The incisions are marked

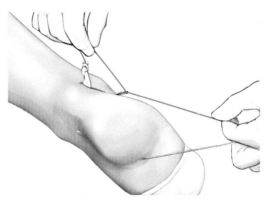

Fig. 15.3 The surgeon is preparing to pass the peroneus tendon through the hole drilled in the calcaneum

15.4 Postoperative Care

Patients are discharged within 24 hours of operation, with the advice to bear weight on the metatarsal heads of the operated foot as tolerated, using elbow crutches. The cast is removed 2 weeks postoperatively, and instructions are given to wear a commercially available removable boot. Proprioception, inversion and eversion exercises and active plantar flexion were recommended, but dorsiflexion was avoided. Patients were permitted to progress gradually to full weight-bearing, generally, by the end of the third week.

After 6 weeks, isometric and concentric contractions of the gastrocnemius–soleus complex are allowed. The boot is removed 8 weeks postoperatively, and patients were allowed to bear full weight without walking aids although heel wedges are recommended until the 3 months time point.

15.5 Pearls and Pitfalls

- Care should be taken to avoid iatrogenic injury on the sural nerve, which passes between the site of mobilization within the peroneal sheath and the insertion of the Achilles tendon. Preoperative skin markings of the course of the nerve are recommended to minimize this risk.

- At the distal fibula, the peroneus brevis tendon is flatter, broader and closer to the bone and has a more distal muscle belly than peroneus longus. These characteristics aid identification.
- The insertion of the peroneus brevis tendon tends to be on the dorsum of the fifth metatarsal and may be longer than expected.

References

1. Hepp WR, Blauth W. Repair of defects in the Achilles tendon with the peroneus brevis muscle (In German). Arch Orthop Trauma Surg. 1978;91:195–200.
2. Maffulli N, Spiezia F, Longo UG, et al. Less-invasive reconstruction of chronic Achilles tendon ruptures using a peroneus brevis tendon transfer. Am J Sports Med. 2010;38:2304–12.
3. Maffulli N, Longo UG, Gougoulias N, et al. Sport injuries: a review of outcomes. Br Med Bull. 2011;97:47–80.
4. Maffulli N, Spiezia F, Pintore E, et al. Peroneus brevis tendon transfer for reconstruction of chronic tears of the Achilles tendon: a long-term follow-up study. J Bone Joint Surg. 2012;94-A:901–5.
5. Miskulin M, Miskulin A, Klobucar H, et al. Neglected rupture of the Achilles tendon treated with peroneus brevis transfer: a functional assessment of 5 cases. J Foot Ankle Surg. 2005;44:49–56.
6. Perez Teuffer A. Traumatic rupture of the Achilles tendon: reconstruction by transplant and graft using the lateral peroneus brevis. Orthop Clin North Am. 1974;5:89–93.
7. Turco VJ, Spinella AJ. Achilles tendon ruptures–peroneus brevis transfer. Foot Ankle. 1987;7:253–9.

Ipsilateral Free Semitendinosus Tendon Graft with Interference Screw Fixation

Rocco Aicale, Domiziano Tarantino, Francesco Oliva, Michael R. Carmont, and Nicola Maffulli

16.1 Indication and Diagnosis

The aim of treatment for chronic tears of the Achilles tendon is to minimise and relieve symptoms and improve function. Surgery aims to restore tendon continuity. However, the stumps of the non-healed tendon can be atrophic, retracted and separated by a gap too large for end-to-end repair even following mobilisation. It is not usual

R. Aicale • D. Tarantino
Department of Musculoskeletal Disorders,
School of Medicine and Surgery, University of Salerno,
Salerno, Italy
e-mail: aicale17@gmail.com;
domiziano22@gmail.com

F. Oliva
Department of Orthopaedics and Traumatology,
University of Rome "Tor Vergata", School of Medicine,
Viale Oxford 81, 00133 Rome, Italy

M.R. Carmont
Department of Trauma & Orthopaedic Surgery,
Princess Royal Hospital, Shrewsbury, UK

Telford Hospital NHS Trust, Shropshire, UK
e-mail: mcarmont@hotmail.com

N. Maffulli (✉)
Queen Mary University of London,
Barts and the London School of Medicine and Dentistry,
Centre for Sports and Exercise Medicine,
Mile End Hospital, 275 Bancroft Road,
London E1 4DG, UK

Department of Musculoskeletal Disorders,
School of Medicine and Surgery, University of Salerno,
Salerno, Italy
e-mail: n.maffulli@qmul.ac.uk

for patients with significant comorbidities to have chronic ruptures to have large gaps (>6 cm) between the tendon ends. Many reconstruction procedures have been proposed, including turndown flaps, tendon transfers, tendon grafts or augmentation with synthetic materials [3], but none of these have been shown to give superior outcomes, making it impossible to draw firm guidelines regarding optimal management [2]. The medical comorbidities that influenced difficulty in initial diagnosis and decision-making may place patients at further risk of wound breakdown with reconstructive procedures. These patients may benefit from minimally invasive techniques to restore tendon continuity and length without excessive tension, recovering isometric plantar flexor strength [5, 6].

Advantages of this minimally invasive technique are that the rupture site is not exposed and skin integrity is preserved, minimising the chance of wound breakdown and postoperative infection. The distal incision allows tendon adherence and scar tissue to be released from the distal stump, and the posterior calcaneal tuberosity is removed to prevent impingement on the calcaneum.

An autologous ipsilateral semitendinosus tendon graft is longer and stronger than an autologous ipsilateral gracilis tendon and is easy to harvest, although it can lead to some weakness during sprinting and deep flexion. Patients with Achilles tendon ruptures tend not to notice the weakness following hamstring harvest, and the

© ESSKA 2017
H. Thermann et al. (eds.), *The Achilles Tendon*, DOI 10.1007/978-3-662-54074-9_16

tendon can regenerate in 70% of patients by 8–12 months [1, 7]. There is no loss of functional toe plantar flexion and eversion associated with local tendon transfer of flexor digitorum longus, flexor hallucis longus and peroneus brevis transfer.

The free hamstring graft is passed into a calcaneum bone tunnel and stabilised using an interference screw. This fixation could potentially be stronger than the stump-graft tenodesis, owing to the greater vascularity of the cancellous calcaneal bone, compared to a degenerate stump or one that has already lead to non-healing [4].

Disadvantages include the learning curve and technically demanding nature of minimally invasive reconstruction, the limited exposure of the proximal tendon and the use of a posterior popliteal fossa incision for graft harvest.

Contraindications to reconstruction using hamstring graft include diabetes, vascular diseases and previous hamstring harvest of the semitendinosus tendon. The consent process should include discussion that if adhesion release is not possible as a minimally invasive procedure, an open procedure may have to be performed, with a change in risk profile. In addition, patients should be warned of the risk of sural nerve injury, which could result in transient, occasionally permanent, sensory loss to the outer aspect of the foot and ankle [8].

16.2 Operative Setup

Surgery is performed under spinal or general anaesthesia. The patient is placed prone with both feet dangling from the edge of the operating table. The tourniquet is positioned as high as possible up the thigh, exsanguination of the limb is performed in a routine fashion, and the tourniquet is inflated to 300 mmHg. After skin prepping in the usual fashion, sterile drapes are applied.

16.3 Surgical Technique

Anatomical landmarks are palpated: the tendon defect, the distal and proximal tendon stumps and the superior posterolateral corner of the calcaneum (Fig. 16.1). Through a transverse 2 cm incision over the medial aspect of the popliteal fossa, the semitendinosus tendon is harvested and prepared at its proximal and distal ends with No. 1 Vicryl (Ethicon, Edinburgh, Scotland) whip sutures. A 3 cm longitudinal incision is performed 2 cm proximal and just medial to the palpable end of the proximal stump. Once the proximal Achilles tendon stump has been freed from all peritendinous adhesions, surrounding fibrotic and scar tissues, it is mobilised. The macroscopically evident healthy tendon is exposed, and the stump is delivered through the wound and trimmed to the healthy tendon (Fig. 16.2).

Next, a 2.5 cm longitudinal incision is made 2 cm distal and just lateral to the lateral margin of the distal stump, taking care to be close to the lateral border of the Achilles tendon and prevent damage to the sural nerve. After removal of adhesions from the distal stump, it is left inside underneath the skin, not exposed from the wound. The Kager's space and the postero-superior corner of the calcaneum are exposed distally, allowing to palpate the Achilles tendon consistency and follow the tendon to the postero-superior corner of the calcaneum (Fig. 16.3). An osteotomy of the postero-superior corner of the calcaneum is then performed using an oscillating saw, paying attention to remove residual bony spurs, which could impinge against the new, reconstructed Achilles tendon (Fig. 16.4). After having drilled the calcaneum from dorsal to plantar with a Beath pin inclined at about 45° to the horizontal, a 7 mm cannulated headed reamer is used to drill a bone tunnel through which the double-stranded semitendinosus tendon graft will be passed. Then, a loop of Ethibond is passed in the eyelet of the Beath pin and left in situ (Fig. 16.5).

The semitendinosus tendon graft is passed through a medial-to-lateral small incision in the proximal stump and secured at the entry and exit points using 2-0 Vicryl (Polyglactin 910 braided absorbable suture; Johnson & Johnson, Brussels,

Belgium) stitches (Fig. 16.6). Once the two ends of the semitendinosus tendon are transported distally, passing underneath the intact skin, the Beath pin is pulled to allow the graft to be shuttled through the bone tunnel (Fig. 16.7). Tensioning the graft from the plantar surface of the foot and keeping the ankle in maximal plantar flexion, a guide wire is used to place a 7 mm by 20 mm or a 7 mm by 25 mm metallic or bioabsorbable interference screw which fixes the graft to the calcaneum (Fig. 16.8). A 2-0 Vicryl

(Polyglactin 910 braided absorbable suture; Johnson & Johnson, Brussels, Belgium) is used to suture the semitendinosus tendon to the distal stump of the Achilles tendon. After thorough irrigation with normal saline, the skin incisions are sutured (2.0 Vicryl suture or 3.0 Biosyn, Tyco Health Care, Norwalk, CT), and Steri-Strips (3 M Health Care, St. Paul, MN) are applied. A below-knee weight-bearing synthetic cast is applied with the foot in maximal plantar flexion.

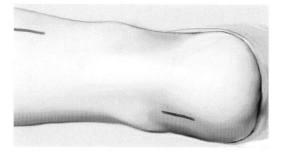

Fig. 16.1 Palpable landmarks include the tendon defect, the distal and proximal tendon stumps and the superior posterolateral corner of the calcaneum

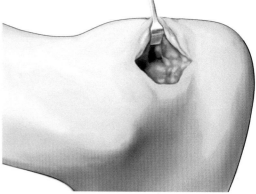

Fig. 16.3 A 2.5 cm longitudinal incision is made 2 cm distal and just lateral to the lateral margin of the distal stump, adhesions are debrided, and care is taken to avoid iatrogenic injury to the sural nerve. The Kager's space and the postero-superior corner of the calcaneum are exposed distally

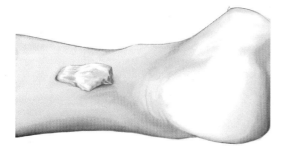

Fig. 16.2 A 3 cm longitudinal incision is performed 2 cm proximal and just medial to the palpable end of the proximal stump. The tendon is debrided to healthy tissue

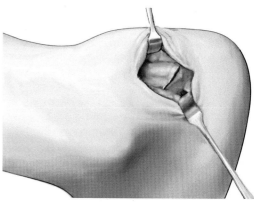

Fig. 16.4 An osteotomy of the postero-superior corner of the calcaneum is then performed using an oscillating saw, paying attention to remove residual bony spurs

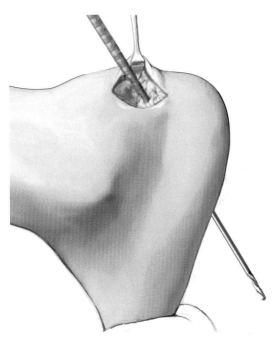

Fig. 16.5 The calcaneal tunnel is drilled from dorsal to plantar direction at 45° using a 7 mm cannulated reamer

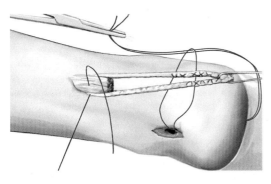

Fig. 16.6 The semitendinosus tendon graft is passed through a medial-to-lateral small incision in the proximal stump and secured at the entry and exit points using a suture

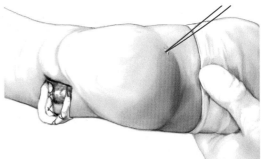

Fig. 16.7 The two ends of the semitendinosus tendon are transported distally, passing underneath the intact skin using a Beath pin to pull the ends through the bone tunnel

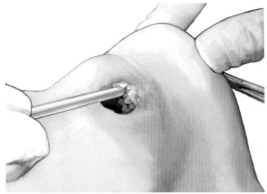

Fig. 16.8 Tensioning the graft from the plantar surface of the foot and keeping the ankle in maximal plantar flexion, a guide wire is used to place an interference screw into the calcaneal tunnel

16.4 Post-operative Care

Rehabilitation is based on gaining proprioception with weight-bearing, early plantar flexion of the ankle, inversion and eversion exercises and the wearing of a protective brace.

Patients are permitted to weight-bear on the metatarsal heads as tolerated using elbow crutches, with the knee flexed. Short walks should be taken at least 5 minutes per hour, and the patient must keep the leg elevated for the first two postoperative weeks, taking care to perform exercise of active flexion and extension of the hallux and toes, isometric of calf muscles and toes, straight leg raises and active flexion and extension of the knee.

At 2 weeks, the cast is removed, and an Aircast boot with five heel wedges (XP Walker, DJO Ltd., Guilford, England, UK) is applied. Proprioception, ankle plantar flexion, inversion and eversion exercises are started. Dorsiflexion and stretching are forbidden, but patients are allowed to full weight-bear with the boot in situ. One heel wedge is removed every 2 weeks, and the boot is taken off after 6 weeks, when only two wedges are left in the boot. Active heel raises are allowed after removal of the boot.

16.5 Pearls, Tips and Pitfalls

- Inadequate exposure and traction of the proximal tendon stump must be treated enlarging the relevant surgical wound.
- Malpositioning or breaking or loosening or mobilisation of the screw must be resolved with removal of the screw and using a larger one.
- Inadequate tension of the fixation requires a revision. Calcaneal fractures must be treated with an open reduction and internal fixation. Infection must be treated with antibiotics.
- Restricted joint motion of the ankle requires early passive and active motion supervised by a physiotherapist.
- Re-ruptures, although rare, require a revision: we have not experienced one such complication. Damage to the sural nerve and wound complications can occur.

References

1. Ferretti A, Conteduca F, Morelli F, Masi V. Regeneration of the semitendinosus tendon after its use in anterior cruciate ligament reconstruction: a histologic study of three cases. Am J Sports Med. 2002;30:204–7.
2. Hadi M, Yung J, Cooper L, Costa M, Maffulli N. Surgical management of chronic ruptures of the Achilles tendon remains unclear: a systematic review of management options. Br Med Bull. 2013;108:95–114.
3. Longo UG, Lamberti A, Maffulli N, Denaro V. Tendon augmentation grafts: a systematic review. Br Med Bull. 2010;94:165–88.
4. Maffulli N, Longo UG, Spiezia F, Denaro V. Free hamstrings tendon transfer and interference screw fixation for less invasive reconstruction of chronic avulsions of the Achilles tendon. Knee Surg Sports Traumatol Arthrosc. 2010;18:269–73.
5. Maffulli N, Del Buono A, Spieza F, Maffulli GD, Longo UG, Denaro V. Less invasive semitendinosus tendon graft augmentation for the reconstruction of chronic tears of the Achilles tendon. Am J Sports Med. 2013;41(4):865–71.
6. Padanilam TG. Chronic Achilles tendon ruptures. Foot Ankle Clin. 2009;14:711–28.
7. Papandrea P, Vulpiani MC, Ferretti A, Conteduca F. Regeneration of the semitendinosus tendon harvested for anterior cruciate ligament reconstruction. Evaluation using ultrasonography. Am J Sports Med. 2000;28:556–61.
8. Wong J, Barrass V, Maffulli N. Quantitative review of operative and nonoperative management of achilles tendon ruptures. Am J Sports Med. 2002;30:565–75.

Endoscopic-Assisted Free Graft Technique with Semi-T Transfer

Hajo Thermann and Christoph Becher

17.1 Indication and Diagnosis

Chronic rupture of the Achilles tendon is commonly a result of a misdiagnosed or neglected acute rupture [1]. Severe intratendineal degenerations with either thickening or thinning of the scar tendon tissue can be observed. The patients feel pain, which is refractory to conservative measures.

Generally, chronic ruptures may show a wide range of impairment. Commonly, a lack of power during "push-off" is present ranging from complete lack of power and failure to raise the heel to a lack of power to stand on toes with maximum plantar flexion. Clinical examination shows an increased dorsiflexion compared to the opposite side, often by 5° or more. Magnetic resonance imaging (MRI) often shows severe degenerative changes and increased signal intensity with partial fluid accumulation in the T2 sequences.

In ruptures with a large gap after debridement of >5 cm, a tendon transfer is necessary [2]. To minimize the risk of soft tissue complications, an endoscopic-assisted approach with a free semi-tendinosus tendon graft appears to be a reasonable operative treatment option. This technique is also suitable for massive defects. The advantage compared with FHL (flexor hallucis longus transfer) is no loss of big toe push-off, especially as the power of plantar flexion is already compromised.

(Creeping) infections need to be completely debrided (sometimes with a second look debridement) before a reconstruction of the tendon (in severe cases after 4–6 weeks) can be performed. In cases of severe arteriovenous occlusive disease, the indication should be very close together and a tourniquet should not be applied.

17.2 Operative Setup

The setup for chronic ruptures is identical to that for the endoscopic treatment of midportion Achilles tendinopathy (see Chap. 8).

Since considerable adhesions are usually present, especially in cases with prior operative treatment, 3.2 mm punches and a normal, stable scissor should be available in order to release the scar tissue.

Special care must be taken not to get into area of the sural nerve, the peripheral lateral arterial vascularization, and the anterior neurovascular bundle.

We recommend to apply fibrin glue (e.g., Tissucol 5 ml) after tendon reconstruction, and if there is the possibility for application, a PRP product, a centrifuge, and appropriate syringe are to be available.

H. Thermann (✉) • C. Becher
International Center of Hip, Knee and Foot Surgery,
ATOS Clinic Heidelberg, Heidelberg, Germany
e-mail: thermann@atos.de; becher.chris@web.de

© ESSKA 2017
H. Thermann et al. (eds.), *The Achilles Tendon*, DOI 10.1007/978-3-662-54074-9_17

17.3   Surgical Technique

The portals are created proximal and distal at the ends of the defect area (Fig. 17.1). The subcutaneous soft tissue is spread with a mosquito clamp along the dorsal portion of the tendon to create a space for endoscopy. In some cases, the use of a stable scissor is necessary for the release of scar tissue. The release is carried out from both the proximal and the distal incision. The arthroscope is inserted through the proximal incision and a 3.8 mm shaver from the distal incision. By triangulation, the shaver is brought directly into the surgical field (see Chap. 8).

In accordance with the MRI, substantial defects with partly hemorrhages and degenerative areas are visible after debridement of the peritendineum. A complete debridement of the degenerative areas has to be performed irrespective of how much tendon needs to be removed (Fig. 17.2). Care must be taken not to lacerate the side branch of the fibular nerve as well as the nearby lying sural nerve on the lateral side as well as the tibial artery with its branches and the tibial nerve on the medial side, respectively.

To harvest the ipsilateral semitendinosus tendon, a transverse incision is made slightly medial to the palpable tendon proximal to the popliteal fossa (Fig. 17.3). The tendon is exposed and dissected from the surrounding tissue and vinculae. The tendon is detached with a common tendon stripper (Fig. 17.4), and the ends of the tendon are prepared with a whipstitch (FiberWire®, Arthrex GmbH, München) in the usual fashion.

For the tendon transfer, a framewise suture using a FiberTape (FiberTape®, Arthrex GmbH, München) to secure the tendon transfer is performed first (Fig. 17.5) by positioning the foot in equinus position. This can also be performed transcalcanear if the remaining distal tendon stump is too short.

A small channel is now created from medial to lateral through the distal tendon stump close to the calcaneus by using an Ellis clamp. The tendon transplant is pulled with the clamp through the distal stump and fixed to the aponeurosis with FiberWire® sutures in Krackow technique. The transplant is then pulled proximally with an awl and the medial end pulled through the proximal tendon aponeurosis to the lateral side and the lateral end to the medial side, respectively. With the foot in maximum plantar flexion, the graft is fixed to the proximal aponeurosis as performed distally with Krackow sutures (Fig. 17.5). For the proximal reconstruction, the portals have to be slightly lengthened.

A PRP product is injected under visual control in the reconstructed areas. Sealing of the entire debrided area with fibrin glue in the sense of "tubulization" is performed under arthroscopic view. A 8 mm drain should be introduced and the incisions closed in common fashion.

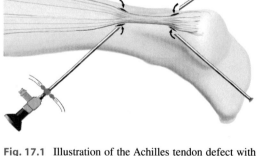

Fig. 17.1 Illustration of the Achilles tendon defect with the four incisions for the endoscopic-assisted tendon free graft technique medial and lateral to the Achilles tendon

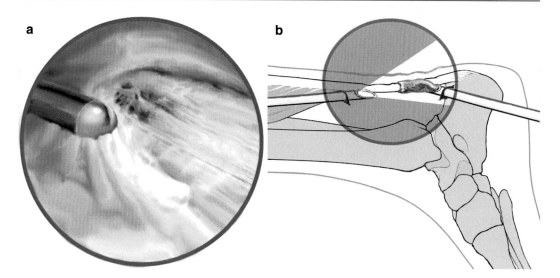

Fig. 17.2 (**a**) Endoscopic debridement of the degenerative areas in chronic ruptures. (**b**) Endoscopic release of the proximal and distal tendon stumps to recreate a functional gastroc-soleus AT unit in defect/infect situation

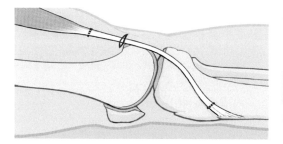

Fig. 17.3 To harvest the ipsilateral semitendinosus tendon, a transverse incision is made slightly medial to the palpable tendon proximal to the popliteal fossa

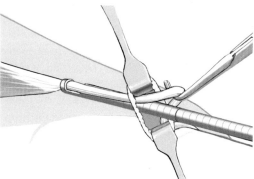

Fig. 17.4 The tendon is detached with a common tendon stripper

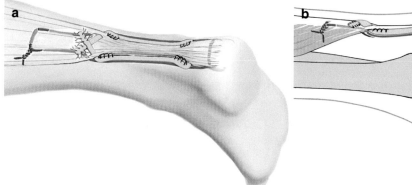

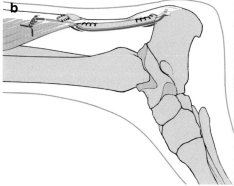

Fig. 17.5 Final result of free graft technique with semi-T transfer. A framewise suture is used to secure the tendon transfer. (**a**) Dorsal view. (**b**) Sagittal view

17.4   Postoperative Care

After application of the wound dressing with cotton wool fixed with an elastic bandage, a prefabricated cardboard splint is applied in equinus position. Moderate movement exercises from 5° to 10° plantar flexion can start from the second/third day as tolerated by pain and swelling.

Thereafter, mild exercise in the form of a "moderate motion" are performed in plantar flexion, thus preventing the scarring of the tendon and allowing early gliding of the tendon. Lymphatic drainage and physiotherapy with motion exercises of the ankle, especially stretching the flexor chain in plantar flexion, are added.

With good wound and swelling conditions, full weight bearing is allowed in the boot (Vario-Stabil, Orthotech GmbH, 82131 Gauting-Stockdorf, Germany). After 6 weeks and ultrasound control, the patient can proceed with the physical therapy and the muscle strengthening (only in plantar flexion!) in case of good graft regeneration. High insoles (2 cm) have to remain for at least another 6 weeks in normal shoes. Uncertain (elderly) patients should wear the boot for another 2 weeks without the plastic "strap-in." This allows a weaning from the protection and is important from a psychological perspective.

17.5   Pearls and Pitfalls

- The additionally used frame suture (FiberTape) acts as a stress bypass for the tendon transplant.
- The FiberTape is tightened in full plantar flexion to have a maximal pull on the proximal gastroc-soleus-Achilles complex.
- For the FiberTape transcalcanear suture, the drill hole should not be too far anterior in the posterior calcaneus to prevent changes in the biomechanics.
- The lateral proximal incision should be enlarged to prevent irritation of the sural nerve.
- After suturing into the aponeurosis, the redundant ends of the tendon transfer should be removed.

References

1. Maffulli N, Ajis A, Longo UG, Denaro V. Chronic rupture of tendo Achillis. Foot Ankle Clin. 2007;12(4):583–96.
2. Myerson MS. Achilles tendon ruptures. Instr Course Lect. 1999;48:219–30.

Endoscopic Flexor Hallucis Longus Tendon Transfer

18

Michael R. Carmont, Jordi Vega, Jorge Batista, and Nuno Corte-Real

18.1 Indication and Diagnosis

Numerous papers report on reconstruction and augmentation of the Achilles tendon using flexor hallucis longus (FHL) tendon transfer as an open surgical technique. Although good outcomes are shown [1], there are risks of infection and wound breakdown.

M.R. Carmont (✉)
The Department of Orthopaedic Surgery,
Princess Royal Hospital, Shrewsbury, UK

Telford Hospital NHS Trust, Shropshire, UK
e-mail: mcarmont@hotmail.com

J. Vega, MD
Foot and Ankle Unit, Hospital Quirón Barcelona,
Barcelona, Spain

Laboratory of Arthroscopic and Surgical Anatomy,
Department of Pathology and Experimental
Therapeutics (Human Anatomy Unit),
University of Barcelona, Barcelona, Spain
e-mail: jordivega@hotmail.com

J. Batista, MD
Centro artroscópico Jorge Batista SA (CAJB),
Av. Pueyrredón 2446 CABA Zi Code,
1119 Buenos Aires, Argentina

Department of Orthopedic Surgery and Sport Medicine,
Brandsen, 805 CABA, Argentina
e-mail: jbatista20@hotmail.com

N. Corte-Real, MD
Orthopaedic Surgery Department,
Hospital de Cascais, Alcabideche, Portugal
e-mail: nc-r@sapo.pt

The greatest increases in incidence of Achilles tendon rupture currently occur in those of 60 years of age. Patients in this age group and those with comorbidities such as diabetes mellitus and peripheral vascular disease and those taking steroids and smokers may have initially received nonoperative treatment with progression to non-healing. Patients may also have a neglected presentation and healing with either tendon elongation or gaping or have sustained a tendon re-rupture. The absence of healing means that this posterior checkrein is lost, permitting ankle hyper-dorsiflexion. The eccentric contraction of the gastrocsoleus complex during terminal stance becomes weak in addition to reduced strength during push-off, and patients commonly report an altered gait, with a visible limp, and balance problems.

In patients, particularly the older population, endoscopic tendon transfer may offer an alternative technique to minimize wound complications [2, 3]. Some authors use this technique in young active patients but this needs further validation. There are many advantages to using FHL transfer rather than transfer of flexor digitorum longus or peroneus brevis. While all of these tendons are in phase or synergy to the Achilles tendon, the FHL is the largest and strongest of these tendons, contributing 3.6% to plantar flexion strength. The FHL is also close and in line with the Achilles tendon so a transfer does not cross the neurovascular bundle. The specific transfer of FHL, as opposed to FDL, minimizes the risk of iatrogenic

© ESSKA 2017
H. Thermann et al. (eds.), *The Achilles Tendon*, DOI 10.1007/978-3-662-54074-9_18

nerve injury. Additionally the vascular low-lying muscle belly of FHL is thought to bring increased perfusion to the compromised Achilles tendon. Transfer of the FHL has the advantage that it does not alter the balance to the ankle joint but on formal testing it does reduce interphalangeal joint flexion strength; however, patients tend to not appreciate this weakness.

In initial open FHL transfers, the tendon was tenodesed to the tendinous portion of the Achilles tendon at the insertion; however, over the last 5 years, reconstructions have anchored grafts and transferred tendons into the calcaneum using a bone tunnel and interference fit screw. The aim of the tendon transfer is to position the FHL as close as possible to the insertion of the Achilles to provide the optimal biomechanical action of the transferred tendon. The anatomical insertion of the tendon is the ideal placement; however, in cases where the FHL is used to augment a minimally invasive repair following rupture, the insertion site should be preserved. The calcaneal tunnel should be targeted as posteriorly as possible to gain maximal biomechanical benefit. The tunnel direction from supero-medial to infero-lateral exits away from the weight-bearing surface. The FHL should be passed into the tunnel so that the low muscular portion of the musculo-tendinous junction of the FHL is level with the tunnel aperture. Remembering that the calcaneum may be osteoporotic, a screw size 1–2 mm greater than the tunnel size can be used, although there is a risk of posterior calcaneal wall blowout. Other risks of surgery include iatrogenic risks of tibial nerve and posterior tibial artery injury. Endoscopic surgery could be considered to pose a higher risk of iatrogenic injury, although the technique offers better indirect vision in the hands of an experienced arthroscopic surgeon than attempting to perform the harvest through a small open incision.

Over time the transferred FHL has been noted to hypertrophy by 15% in 80% of patients. Other series have reported outcomes at 27 months following reconstruction of an ATRS of 70 and a 52% hypertrophy of the FHL. It is also possible that the gastrocsoleus is to regain activity following transfer.

Endoscopic FHL transfer offers an acceptable low-risk method to reconstruct the Achilles tendon with minimal wound risks and to optimize gait and function in the low/moderate demand population.

18.2   Operative Setup

A laminar flow operating theater is preferable. Popliteal peripheral nerve blockade or spinal/general anesthesia rather than local anesthetic field infiltration is required.

The patient is positioned in the lateral recovery/extended lateral position, with the operated side down. The thigh tourniquet should be applied prior to turning. Care must be taken to ensure that the lower shoulder is flexed to prevent venous compression. The pelvis is tilted and the operated lower hip is externally rotated. The ankle may rest on a supportive bolster. The opposite hip and knee are flexed, and a supportive strap may be applied around the knee to support the pelvis reducing rotational forces on the lumbar spine.

Two applications of 2% chlorhexidine skin preparation are used up to the tourniquet. A knee arthroscopy drape with a fluid collection bag can be applied with one sleeve around the calf and another around the mid-foot secured with a towel clip.

18.3 Surgical Technique

The postero-superior calcaneal tubercle is identified using a posterolateral hindfoot arthroscopy portal together with a high postero-medial portal (Fig. 18.1). Standard endoscopic approach to the posteromedial side of the ankle is performed to identify the FHL tendon and the fibro-osseous sheath. Care should be taken to preserve as much of the retrocalcaneal fat pad as possible.

An accessory posterolateral portal is inserted just posterior to the peroneal sheath, and the scope is introduced to allow indirect vision down the axis of the calcaneum toward the postero-superior calcaneal tubercle and the Achilles tendon. Using a 12 fluted barrel bur, the tubercle is debrided to provide the entry point for the drilling of the calcaneal tunnel.

With the ankle and metatarsophalangeal joint in full flexion, the FHL tendon is visualized on the medial aspect of the ankle and subtalar joints before it enters the FHL sheath (Fig. 18.2). A locking suture is passed through the tendon of FHL as distally as possible via the posteromedial portal (Fig. 18.3). This suture is used to apply tension to the FHL tendon so that all residual slack tendon passes out of the sheath; alternatively an arthroscopic grasper may be used to apply tension to the FHL (Fig. 18.4). This allows a scalpel or arthroscopy scissors to cut the FHL as distally as possible under arthroscopic vision to avoid iatrogenic injury (Fig. 18.5). The FHL tendon can then be delivered from the higher pos-teromedial portal to allow a whip suture to be applied (Fig. 18.6).

The FHL tendon is then secured into the calcaneum using either the biotenodesis or interference screw technique. For the biotenodesis technique, a 5 mm tunnel is made with a reamer to a depth of 15–20 mm. A loop is used to hold a 5.5 mm screw on the tendon approximately 20 mm from the FHL musculotendinous junction. The introducer is then tapped into position and the biotenodesis screw advanced into position (Fig. 18.7).

Using an interference screw, the ankle is held in full plantar flexion; a Beath pin is passed through the posteromedial portal onto the distal calcaneum under visualization via the Acc PL portal. The Beath passing pin is directed infero-laterally so that it emerges from the lateral aspect of the heel (Fig. 18.8). A 6 mm reamer is then used to create the calcaneal tunnel. The Beath pin is then used to pass a pull-through suture through the calcaneal tunnel to pass the ends of the FHL tendon whip suture through the calcaneal tunnel.

With the ankle in full plantar flexion, the FHL is pulled into the calcaneal tunnel until the muscle belly of FHL is at the level of the tunnel aperture. The tendon is secured using an interference screw 1–2 mm wider than the calcaneal tunnel under arthroscopic vision. Incisions are closed using subcutaneous Vicryl and Monocryl for the skin. Dressings and an anterior plaster of Paris slab are applied and overwrapped with crepe. Alternatively a preformed functional brace can be applied.

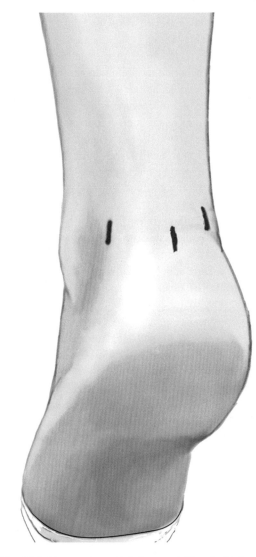

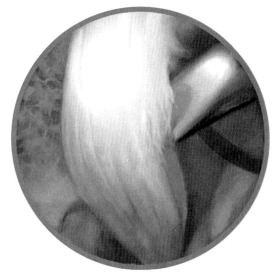

Fig. 18.2 The FHL tendon as it passes into its fibro-osseous sheath

Fig. 18.1 Preoperative portal placement. Note the higher position of the larger posteromedial portal. This permits the FHL tendon to be passed out of the skin for the application of a whip suture and also the antegrade drill passage of the bio-interference screw

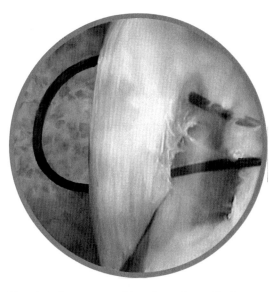

Fig. 18.3 A suture passed into the tendon as distal as possible permits the tendon to be placed under tension as it is harvested, optimizing tendon length and minimizing risk of iatrogenic nerve injury

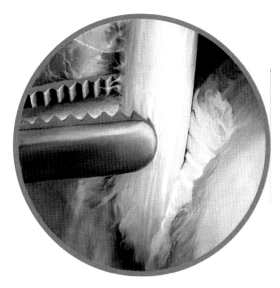

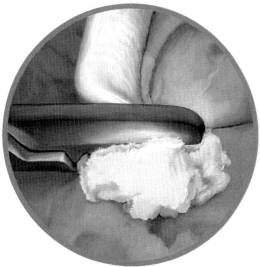

Fig. 18.4 Alternatively the FHL tendon may be grasped using an arthroscopic grasper or hook

Fig. 18.5 The tendon is then cut under arthroscopic vision to minimize the risk of iatrogenic nerve injury

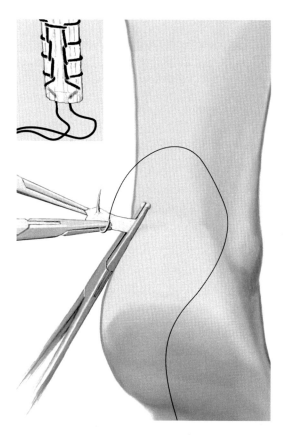

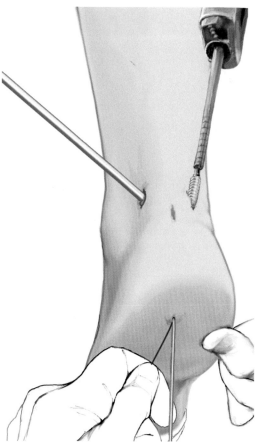

Fig. 18.6 The tendon is then delivered through the posteromedial portal and a whip suture applied

Fig. 18.7 The tendon is passed into the calcaneal tunnel under direct vision so that the musculotendinous portion is at the tunnel aperture using a biotenodesis screw

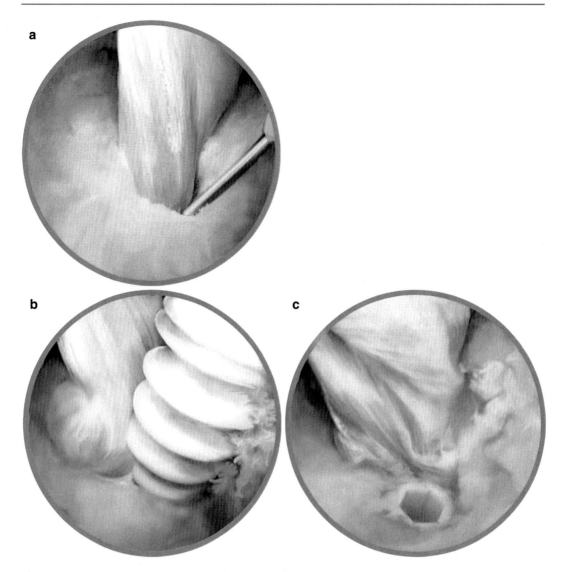

Fig. 18.8 (**a–c**) Endoscopic visualization of the passage of tendon, guide wire, and screw minimizes problems during this part of the procedure

18.4 Postoperative Care

Postoperatively the patient is placed into a functional brace made from synthetic cast material in equinus or a below knee plaster shell. Once the portals have healed, sutures are removed. At 2 weeks, the dorsal shell is continued together with a boot with three heel wedges. Toe-touch weight-bearing uses axillary crutches as tolerated by pain for 4 weeks. Low-molecular-weight heparin is administered for this period. After 4 weeks, progressive weight-bearing is permitted from toe touch to full using the shell and wedged boot. The crutches may be exchanged for elbow crutches.

At the 6 weeks time point, the brace is discontinued and full weight-bearing commenced using a 15 mm heel wedge in the shoe on both feet until the 3 months following transfer. Crutches are usually continued until the patient is comfortable with walking without assistance; typically this is the 2 months time point.

Formal physiotherapy is commenced at 6 weeks with exercises designed to progressively increase the strength and range of motion of the ankle joint. Initially the bilateral standing or seated heel-rises can be initiated to strengthening the calf musculature. The load on the injured leg is progressively increased, and the goal is to be able to achieve a unilateral heel-rise in standing.

Other impairments in the lower extremity should also be addressed, and the aim is for the patient to walk without a limp and have normal push-off during gait within the first 3–5 weeks. Stretching should be avoided and plyometric exercises should only be permitted at the 3 months time point.

No other time guides are recommended after 3 months, and activities including running and jumping can be introduced when the patient has achieved the ability to perform single-leg heel-rises, can walk without a limb, and has good single-leg balance.

18.5 Pearls, Tips, and Pitfalls

- The FHL passing suture should be placed as distally as possible in the tendon before it enters the sheath. This suture and/or an arthroscopic hook can be used to pull the tendon away from the neurovascular bundle allowing it to be cut under arthroscopic clear vision.
- Additional whip sutures should be placed onto the FHL tendon so that maximal traction can be applied to the tendon in the calcaneal tunnel.
- The calcaneal cancellous bone may well be osteoporotic so a screw 1–2 mm greater than the tunnel diameter is recommended.

References

1. Hansen Jr ST. Trauma to the heel cord. In: Jahss MH, editor. Disorders of the foot and ankle. 3rd ed. Philadelphia: WB Saunders; 1991.
2. Goncalves S, Caetano R, Corte-Real N. Salvage Flexor Hallucis Longus transfer for a failed Achilles repair: endoscopic technique. Arthosc Tech. 2015;4(5): 411–6.
3. Lui TH, Chan WC, Maffulli N. Endoscopic Flexor Hallucis Longus tendon transfer for chronic Achilles tendon rupture. Sports Med Arthrosc. 2016;24:38–41.

Part V

Achilles Tendon Lengthening

Minimally Invasive Lengthening of the Achilles Tendon

19

Olof Westin, Jonathan Reading,
Michael R. Carmont, and Jon Karlsson

19.1 Indication and Diagnosis

Gastrocnemius recession is a common treatment for paediatric patients with spastic equinus often due to neurological conditions, e.g. cerebral palsy. Although the literature is expanding, there is still little evidence on which to base treatment recommendations for recession as other orthopaedic problems relating to gastrocnemius recession.

The incidence of gastrocnemius tightness is twice that of the normal population in patients with metatarsalgia, Morton's foot, tibialis posterior insufficiency and plantar fasciitis. Equinus contracture of the ankle has been found in over 10% all diabetic patients.

Gastrocnemius contracture is defined as less than 10 degrees of ankle dorsiflexion with the knee extended compared with when flexed. Tightness to the Achilles tendon complex consisting of the gastrocnemius and soleus occurs when ankle dorsiflexion cannot be achieved with the knee in both flexion and extension (Fig. 19.1). This is a variation of Silfverskiöld's test [1]. This Achilles tendon tightness alters lower limb biomechanics and results in disturbed loading during gait.

There is some convincing evidence to support the use of gastrocnemius recession for the management of isolated foot pain due to midfootforefoot overload syndrome. Some evidence can also be found in the literature for the treatment of non-insertional Achilles tendinopathy.

The aims of treatment are to treat the mechanical aspects of the problem by reducing the tension applied to the Achilles tendon. Physiotherapy programmes aimed at stretching the calf muscles can be instigated, and the use of splints may be beneficial, but frequently there are issues with compliance. Surgery aims to elongate the Achilles tendon, alleviating the tightness whilst maintaining calf muscle strength and function.

Surgical intervention can be applied at all locations along the length of the gastrosoleus-Achilles tendon complex. The complex has been divided into 3 zones based upon the musculotendinous composition of the zone, the extent of lengthening and the stability of the release [3] (Fig. 19.2).

Zone 1: Lengthening within the gastrocnemius-soleus muscle complex, by different amounts, resulting in a stable but limited lengthening. A Baumann release is an intramuscular lengthening consisting of 3 transverse intramuscular tenotomies,

O. Westin • J. Karlsson (✉)
The Department of Orthopaedic Surgery,
Sahlgrenska Academy, University of Gothenburg,
Gothenburg, Sweden
e-mail: olof.westin@gmail.com;
Jon.Karlsson@telia.com

J. Reading • M.R. Carmont
The Department of Orthopaedic Surgery,
Princess Royal Hospital, Shrewsbury, UK

Telford Hospital NHS Trust, Shropshire, UK
e-mail: jonathan_reading@hotmail.com;
mcarmont@hotmail.com

© ESSKA 2017
H. Thermann et al. (eds.), *The Achilles Tendon*, DOI 10.1007/978-3-662-54074-9_19

each <1 mm to a total of 2.1 mm. A Strayer muscle recession by aponeurosis lengthening is performed through a 5 cm incision commenced 2 cm distal to the visible musculotendinous junction and extended proximally. The gastrocnemius tendon is separated from the soleus by blunt dissection and cut transversely under direct vision; the two edges of tendon are left free and not sutured. The Strayer gastrocnemius recession leads to greater lengthening than after the Baumann recession.

Zone 2: Lengthening at the conjoined gastrocnemius aponeurosis and soleus fascia. This is not selective, however stable, and results in a greater lengthening than zone 1 procedures. The Vulpius tenotomy is an inverted V, whereas the Baker tenotomy comprises a tongue in groove gastrocnemius recession. The midline raphe is also released in both procedures. The gap opens slowly and progressively requiring greater force per centimetre compared to zone 3 procedures.

Zone 3: Procedures are performed within the substance of the Achilles tendon and as a result are neither selective nor stable, but lead to greater lengthening. Double and triple tendon hemisections are described by Hoke and White, respectively. The relative instability after zone 3 lengthening and the continued tendency for further lengthening under small loads suggest greater caution. The position in cast, the postoperative rehabilitation and use of post-operative ankle foot orthosis may influence the long-term clinical outcomes.

The advantages of zone 3 procedures are that only small incisions are required since the tendon is relatively superficial and the proximity to the centre of axis of the ankle joint means that a greater amount of dorsiflexion is achieved per amount of lengthening. The amount of lengthening required for a specific degree of fixed equinus is often much less than surgeons estimate. This can be achieved by geometric methods and musculoskeletal modelling. One degree of increased dorsiflexion can be achieved for each 1 mm of tendon lengthening.

Specific complications of minimally invasive Achilles lengthening include calf weakness and calcaneus gait in addition to iatrogenic sural nerve injury. It is usually impossible to correct an excessively long and weak gastrocnemius-soleus complex. Open procedures such as Z elongation take longer operative time and tend to result in greater scarring with increased risk of adhesion formation.

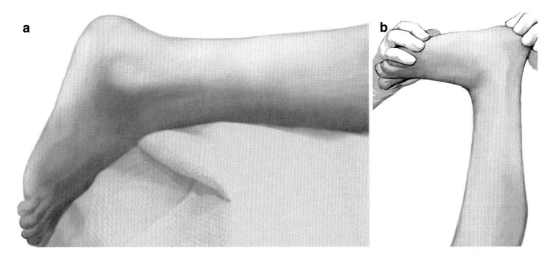

Fig. 19.1 (a, b) Silfverskiöld's test for gastrocnemius contracture with reduced passive ankle dorsiflexion in (a) knee extension compared to (b) knee flexion

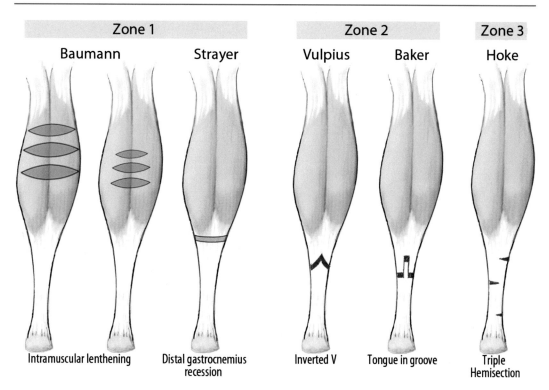

Fig. 19.2 Schematic illustration of the sites and forms of gastrocnemius lengthening

19.2 Operative Setup

A laminar flow operating theatre is preferable. The patient is positioned in the lateral recovery position, with the operated side down. The thigh tourniquet should be applied prior to turning the patient. Care must be taken to ensure that the lower shoulder is flexed to prevent venous compression. The pelvis is tilted and the lower leg to be operated on is externally rotated. The opposite hip and knee are flexed and a supportive strap may be applied around the knee to support the pelvis reducing rotational forces on the lumbar spine.

Alternatively surgeons may prefer to position the patient fully prone. This allows the comparison of Achilles tendon tightness with the non-operated side. Extra assistance for leg elevation during skin preparation and a drape with two leg holes are required if the patient is prone. Two applications of 2% chlorhexidine skin preparation are used up to the tourniquet.

19.3 Surgical Technique

In treatment of symptomatic pes planus, the translational calcaneus osteotomy is performed and stabilized, prior to the Achilles tendon lengthening and then finally a tendon transfer if required. Ankle dorsiflexion compresses the osteotomy whilst stabilization is performed.

Skin marking of the course of the sural nerve is recommended (Fig. 19.3). The nerve typically passes one fingerbreadth distal to the lateral malleolus, midway between the posterior aspect of the lateral malleolus and the lateral side of the Achilles tendon insertion and finally crossing the lateral aspect of the Achilles tendon at 8–10 cm from the insertion to the calcaneus.

For a triple hemisection, three skin incisions are made with the proximal and distal incisions, close to the tendon edge, placed laterally in valgus heels and medially for varus heels. The middle incision is made on the opposite side of the tendon, midway between the other incisions. Blunt dissection of the subcutaneous tissue allows exposure of the fascia cruris and paratenon layers, which can be incised to permit exposure of the tendon. At the proximal incision, care is taken to identify, mobilize and protect the sural nerve (Fig. 19.4).

The tendon is placed under tension by dorsiflexing the ankle, and the tendon is cut at the three sites (Fig. 19.5). The width of transection at each level can gradually be increased whilst forced dorsiflexion is maintained until the tendon elongates to the required length. Lengthening of 1 mm corresponds to 1° of dorsiflexion; therefore, gaping of 3–5 mm at each hemisection results in up to 15° of dorsiflexion.

The separated tendon ends should not be sutured but the subcutaneous and skin sutures are applied. The ankle is placed into a below-knee back slab to maintain ankle dorsiflexion (Fig. 19.6).

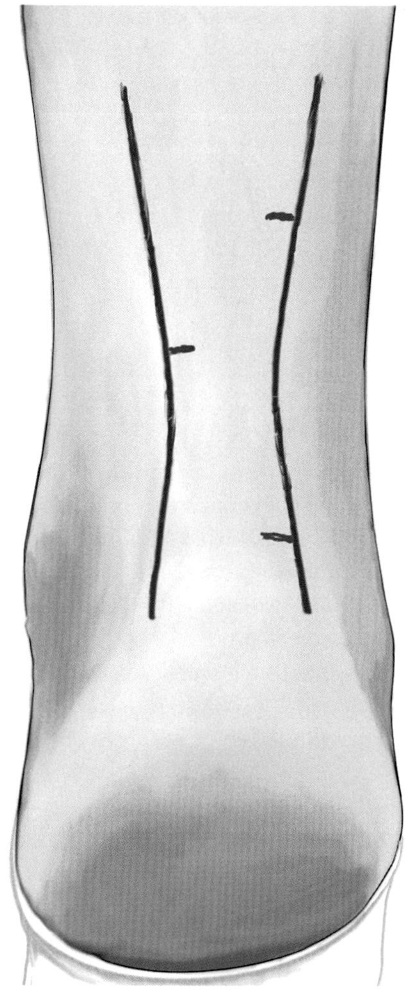

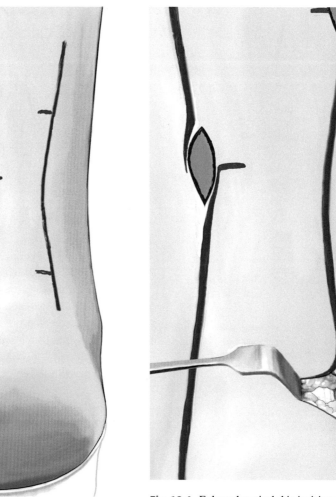

Fig. 19.3 Skin markings of the Achilles tendon, the sural nerve and the position of the triple hemisections

Fig. 19.4 Enlarged vertical skin incisions for the illustration to visualize the edges of the Achilles tendon. The fascia cruris and the paratenon should also be incised

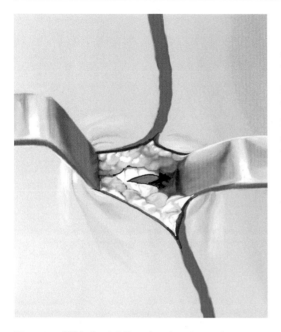

Fig. 19.5 With the Achilles placed under tension, a progressive hemisection is performed until the edge of the Achilles tendon gaps between 2 and 5 mm

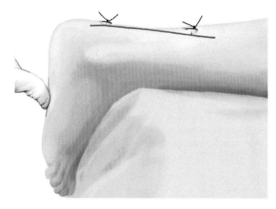

Fig. 19.6 Repeat assessing for heel cord tightness following lengthening shows increased ankle dorsiflexion with the knee in extension

19.4 Post-operative Care

Once the wounds are healed, the back shell may be removed and replaced with an ankle foot orthosis to maintain dorsiflexion. This should be worn for day and night for 6 weeks. Then dorsiflexion, plantar flexion, inversion and eversion exercises should be started and a structured rehabilitation programme initiated.

19.5 Pearls, Tips and Pitfalls

- Gastrocnemius contracture should be assessed before and after concurrent procedures by passive ankle dorsiflexion with the knee in extension and flexion.
- If calcaneal osteotomy is required, this should be performed before heel cord lengthening.
- Hemisection and separation of the Achilles tendon should be performed under direct vision, with the ankle in forced dorsiflexion.

References

1. Cychosz CC, Phisitkul P, Belatti DA, Glazebrook MA, DiGiovanni CW. Gastrocnemius recession for foot and ankle conditions in adults: evidence based recommendations. Foot Ankle Surg. 2015;21:77–85.
2. Silfverskiold N. Reduction of the uncrossed two joint muscles of the leg to one joint muscles in spastic conditions. Acta Chir Scand. 1924;56:315–30.
3. Firth GB, McMullan M, Chin T, Ma F, Selber P, Eizenberg N, Wolfe R, Kerr Graham H. Lengthening of the gastrocsoleus complex. J Bone Joint Surg Am. 2013;95:1489–96.

Gastrocnemius Slide

20

Christoph Becher and Hajo Thermann

20.1 Indication and Diagnosis

A gastrocnemius contracture is characterized by the inability to bend the ankle joint past a neutral position. The diagnosis is made by means of evaluation of the patient's range of dorsiflexion with the knee straight. Many gastrocnemius contractures are subtle, and patients are often asymptomatic since the contracture can be compensated through motion of the midfoot. When making a diagnosis, dorsiflexion is evaluated with the knee both flexed to relax the upper end of the gastrocnemius and extended to tighten it. The foot is hold in a neutral position and locks the talonavicular joint into neutral by means of positioning the foot into slight supination and forefoot adduction preventing motion through the midfoot. Limited dorsiflexion with the knee straight is indicative of a tight gastrocnemius.

If conservative management that includes a calf stretching program and use of orthotics fails, the midfoot capsules have been stretched, and if pronation or lateral peritalar subluxation has degenerated to a pathologic condition, surgery with gastrocnemius lengthening is indicated [1]. Furthermore, the presented technique is very useful as an additional procedure when a gastrocnemius contracture is present (e.g. in total ankle arthroplasty) or created by the procedure (e.g. in open wedge supramalleolar osteotomy). In patients with neurological origin of the contracture, the Achilles tendon should be lengthened.

20.2 Operative Setup

The procedure is usually performed in the prone position with the leg hanging slightly over the table edge unless this position is contraindicated by other procedures performed in the same operation. The other leg is lowered slightly. In order to bring the hind foot in a straight position, a small wedge is placed below the contralateral pelvis. The lower leg and the foot are in a neutral position. The lower leg can also be stabilized with a special elastic pad. Great attention should be paid to prevent pressure damage in the area of the peroneal nerve, sural nerve and the foot. A tourniquet should be used with exsanguination of the leg. General anaesthesia is the most suitable. Antibiotic prophylaxis is recommended by using a third-generation cephalosporin.

C. Becher (✉) • H. Thermann
International Center for Hip-, Knee- and Foot Surgery,
ATOS Clinic Heidelberg, Heidelberg, Germany
e-mail: becher.chris@web.de; thermann@atos.de

© ESSKA 2017
H. Thermann et al. (eds.), *The Achilles Tendon*, DOI 10.1007/978-3-662-54074-9_20

20.3   Surgical Technique

The incision is made horizontally or longitudinally medial to the midline over the distal end of the gastrocnemius (Fig. 20.1) and is usually located over the junction of the middle and distal third of the posterior calf. The saphenous vein and the sural nerve near the midline of the leg should be identified and retracted to the lateral side.

The superficial fascia is separated by a longitudinal or horizontal incision and retracted to expose the distal heads of the medial and lateral gastrocnemius. The deep portions of the gastrocnemius and the soleus fascia are not attached to one another until they meet at the distal end of the gastrocnemius muscle.

Using a scalpel, the gastrocnemius fascia is incised at the lower level leaving the soleus fascia intact (Fig. 20.2). The fascia must be divided completely along with the plantaris tendon on the medial side. With the knee extended, the ankle is positioned first into supination and then into dorsiflexion to slide the gastrocnemius fascia 2–4 cm proximally over the underlying soleus fascia (Fig. 20.3a, b).

The thin fascia overlying the muscle is closed with fine absorbable sutures. The skin is closed in common fashion.

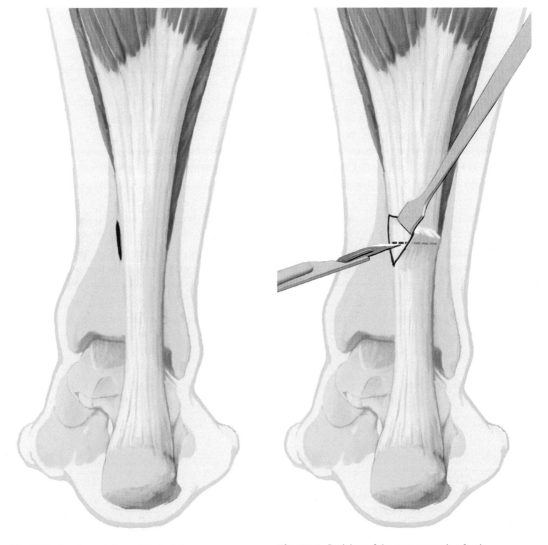

Fig. 20.1 Implementation of the incision

Fig. 20.2 Incision of the gastrocnemius fascia

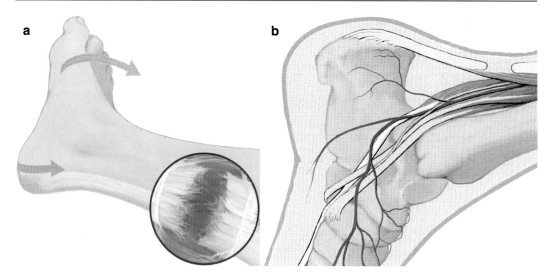

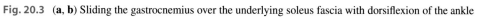

Fig. 20.3 (**a, b**) Sliding the gastrocnemius over the underlying soleus fascia with dorsiflexion of the ankle

20.4   Postoperative Care

After application of the wound dressing with cotton fixed with an elastic bandage, a prefabricated cardboard splint is applied in dorsiflexed position. Movement exercises can start form the second day as tolerated by pain and swelling. Full weight bearing is allowed with the use of a knee-length walker. The walker can be removed after 2–4 weeks. Lymphatic drainage and physiotherapy with motion exercises of the ankle, especially stretching the flexor chain, is added.

20.5   Pearl Tips and Pitfalls

- The splitting of the aponeurosis should be performed step by step with controlled increase of dorsiflexion.

- Care must be taken not to injure the sural nerve and saphenous vein.
- A gastroc slide is only effective if you have a mobile gastrocnemius/soleus-Achilles unit (cave revision surgery).

Reference

1. Hansen ST. Achilles tendon lengthening: gastrocnemius slide. In: Hansen ST, editor. Functional reconstruction of the foot and ankle. Philadelphia: Lippincott, Williams & Wilkins; 2000. p. 415–7.

Part VI

Achilles Tendon Shortening

Z Shortening of Healed Achilles Tendon Rupture

21

Rocco Aicale, Domiziano Tarantino,
Alessio Giai Via, Francesco Oliva,
and Nicola Maffulli

21.1 Indication and Diagnosis

Achilles tendon ruptures are common, but the correct diagnosis may be missed in up to 20% of patients at initial presentation [1].

Following a rupture, the Achilles tendon may still heal. The healing tissue is comprised of tenocytes and fibroblasts and then matures into scar tissue [2]. The new scar tissue is weaker than the original tendon and elongates with time, resulting in weakness of plantar flexion strength [3].

Following rupture, the tendon ends may separate by several centimeters, leaving a large gap which will stay empty, or be filled up by fibrous tissue. At surgery, resection of this fibrous scar tissue may leave a large defect, and, despite mobilization techniques of the proximal musculotendinous junction, the gap may not be adequately bridged to allow end-to-end repair [3, 4].

In some patients, a chronic rupture of the Achilles tendon may heal in continuity, resulting in a lengthened Achilles tendon [5]. The elongated structure must now be shortened or reconstructed to allow some restoration of push-off.

Several techniques have been described for reconstruction of the Achilles tendon [5]. Z lengthening is commonly used for tendon lengthening in patients with equinus contracture of the ankle. Z shortening has been reported for operative shortening of the elongated Achilles tendon following previous rupture [6]. We describe a modification of this technique in the management of chronic ruptures of the Achilles tendon which have healed in continuity but have resulted in an elongated, nonfunctional gastrocsoleus. This technique allows early weight bearing and early active mobilization of the ankle.

The technique described allows close approximation of normal tendon tissue, optimizes the strength of the repair, and minimizes further scar formation and subsequent potential for scar elongation and further weakness of plantar flexion. It has the additional benefit of restoring tendon function without the use of a tendon transfer and its morbidity [5].

R. Aicale, MS-V • D. Tarantino, MS-V
Department of Musculoskeletal Disorders,
School of Medicine and Surgery,
University of Salerno, Salerno, Italy
e-mail: aicale17@gmail.com;
domiziano22@gmail.com

A.G. Via, MD • F. Oliva, MD, PhD
Department of Orthopaedic and Traumatology,
University of Rome "Tor Vergata", School of Medicine,
Viale Oxford 81, 00133 Rome, Italy
e-mail: alessiogiaivia@hotmail.it;
olivafrancesco@hotmail.com

N. Maffulli, MD, MS, PhD, FRCS (Orth) (✉)
Department of Musculoskeletal Disorders,
School of Medicine and Surgery,
University of Salerno, Salerno, Italy

Queen Mary University of London,
Barts and the London School of Medicine and
Dentistry, Centre for Sports and Exercise Medicine,
Mile End Hospital, 275 Bancroft Road,
London E1 4DG, UK
e-mail: n.maffulli@qmul.ac.uk

© ESSKA 2017
H. Thermann et al. (eds.), *The Achilles Tendon*, DOI 10.1007/978-3-662-54074-9_21

21.2   Operative Setup

Skin preparation and sterile drapes are used. A calf tourniquet is applied and inflated to 250 mmHg after exsanguination. Surgery is performed under locoregional anesthesia. Antibiotic preoperative prophylaxis is implemented with first-generation cephalosporins. Postoperative thrombosis prophylaxis is recommended according to patients' risk stratification.

The patient is placed prone with the ankles clear of the operating table. The prone position allows excellent access to the affected area.

21.3   Surgical Technique

Following preoperative skin marking, a medial gently curvilinear incision is made. This permits adequate exposure of the Achilles tendon and identification of the sural nerve. Peritendinous adherences to the superficial tissues are frequently present and released with a scissor (Fig. 21.1). The tendon is macroscopically intact, having healed in continuity, although it is elongated. Macroscopically, it may be possible to detect healthy areas of the tendon, whereas the scar tissue lacks fibrous continuity and is white and translucent. Once the area of the normal tendon has been established, it is mobilized from the fascia of flexor hallucis longus. In these patients, the Kager's triangle is greatly reduced, and often the Achilles tendon lies directly on the fascia of the flexor hallucis longus.

A longitudinal split is made through the length of the healed scar area extending from normal tendon proximally through the healed area into the normal tendon distally. The opposing halves of the tendon are released on opposing sides in a Z shape (Figs. 21.2 and 21.3). With the ankle held in full plantar flexion, the opposing strands of the shortened Z are resected to leave enough tissue to adequately approximate opposing tendon ends with the ankle in full plantar flexion. If necessary, the tendon can be debulked (Fig. 21.4).

The approximated transverse halves are then sutured using a modified Kessler suture, further increasing the strength of the repair (Fig. 21.5). A longitudinal running suture is then used to secure both halves of the tendon using Number 1 Maxon (Tyco Healthcare, Norwalk, CT) (Fig. 21.6). Using tissue forceps, the tendon is turned over, and the undersurface of the incision is sutured again using the locking, running Maxon suture. The final knot of Maxon is tied on the under surface of the tendon so that it would not irritate the overlying skin. Care is taken to ensure that the exposed sural nerve is not damaged.

An absorbable suture is used to impart initial strength to the repair itself. As healing progresses and the suture material degrades, progressively greater loads are transmitted to the tendon itself, allowing appropriate physiological healing. Moreover, using absorbable material, the presence of a permanent foreign body which could act as a focus of infection is avoided.

The wound is closed in layers. The wound edges are covered with Steri-Strips (3M Health Care, St Paul, MN), and a Mepore (Molnlycke Health Care, Gothenburg, Sweden) dressing is applied.

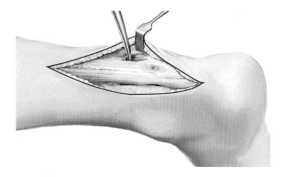

Fig. 21.1 Release of peritendinous adherences to the superficial tissues with a scissor

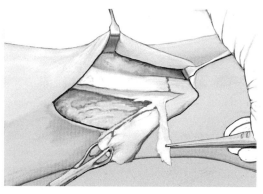

Fig. 21.4 Debulking of the tendon with resection of degenerative tissue

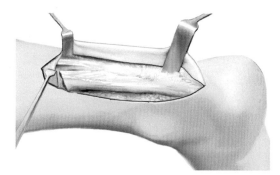

Fig. 21.2 Proximal tendon release to half of the tendon

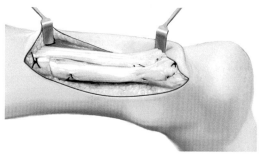

Fig. 21.5 A modified Kessler suture is used to further increase the strength of the repair and secure the approximated transverse halves

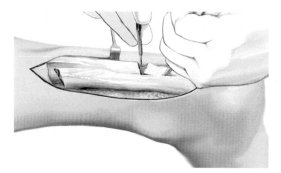

Fig. 21.3 Release in the opposing side in a Z shape

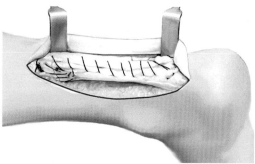

Fig. 21.6 A longitudinal running suture is then used to secure both halves of the tendon

21.4 Postoperative Care

Postoperatively, the patient is allowed to fully weight bear in a bivalved removable synthetic cast in full equinus on the exposed metatarsal heads. Patients are encouraged to perform active flexion and extension of the hallux and toes and to perform isometric exercises of the calf muscles and of the toes. At 2 weeks following surgery, the back shell from the cast is removed, leaving the front shell of the cast secured in place by Velcro straps. This allows active inversion, eversion, and plantar flexion physiotherapy exercises, but prevents dorsiflexion which may damage the repair. During this period of rehabilitation, the patient is permitted to weight bear as comfort allows with the front shell in situ, although full weight bearing rarely occurs on account of balance difficulties and patients usually still require the assistance of a single elbow crutch as this stage. At 6 weeks following surgery, the front shell is removed. A heel raise after removal of the cast is not necessary, and patients are mobilized in an ordinary shoe with the use of a heel lift.

21.5 Pearls Tips and Pitfalls

- The shape of the Z allows overlap of the repair site minimizing local loading and the continuity of the tendon structure minimizes scar tissue formation.

- Z shortening allows wide, close approximation of the tendon without leaving a defect. This will minimize interposed scar tissue between the tendon ends and reduce the risk of further elongation.
- Modified Kessler sutures are used along the transverse cuts of the Z.
- Complications include wound breakdown and sural nerve damage. Careful dissection of the pseudotendon will preserve skin flap thickness to reduce the risk of skin breakdown.
- Full weight bearing following repair is optimal for tendon healing and shortens the time needed for rehabilitation.

References

1. Maffulli N. Clinical tests in sports medicine: more on Achilles tendon. Br J Sports Med. 1996;30(3):250.
2. Sharma P, Maffulli N. Tendon injury and tendinopathy: healing and repair. J Bone Joint Surg Am. 2005; 87(1):187–202.
3. Myerson MS. Achilles tendon ruptures. Instr Course Lect. 1999;48:219–30.
4. Kuwada GT. Classification of tendo Achillis rupture with consideration of surgical repair techniques. J Foot Surg. 1990;29(4):361–5.
5. Maffulli N et al. Chronic rupture of tendo Achillis. Foot Ankle Clin. 2007;12(4):583–96.
6. Cannon LB, Hackney RG. Operative shortening of the elongated defunctioned tendoachillies following previous rupture. J R Nav Med Serv. 2003;89(3): 139–41.

Endoscopically Assisted Mini-open Technique

22

Hajo Thermann and Christoph Becher

22.1 Indication and Diagnosis

Elongation of the Achilles tendon with resulting weakness of plantar flexion strength may be found after a chronic neglected rupture and conservative or operative treatment of an acute rupture.

Typical symptoms include impairment in activities of daily living such as climbing stairs, walking up a hill, or during sports activities due to a loss of power at push-off.

At clinical examination, marked atrophy of the calf muscles is the first sign at inspection. Functional testing may reveal intact plantar flexion. However, single-leg toe raises are impossible to perform or unequivocally diminished in comparison to the unaffected contralateral side. The calf-squeeze test usually produces some motion in the ankle, but less in comparison to the contralateral side. The knee-flexion test in prone position with knees 90° flexed reveals increased passive dorsiflexion in comparison to the contralateral side. On palpation, no gap can be found with variable diameters of the tendon depending on the course of lengthening. Chronic, neglected ruptures usually result in a thin fibrous scar tissue, whereas healed tendons with elongation after operative treatment are usually thickened.

The operative treatment with open z shortening has been shown to be effective in restoration of function [1, 2], although it appears that there is permanent loss of plantar flexion of the gastroc-soleus complex [2]. The open approach implies increased risk of wound breakdown and complications. An arthroscopically assisted mini-open may decrease the risk of wound complications as shown with other minimally invasive techniques for Achilles tendon repair [3].

Indications for the technique described in this article include failed conservative management with extensive training of the gastroc-soleus complex with abovementioned clinical findings. Contraindications are minor functional deficits, high risk for wound complications due to skin alterations after earlier operative treatment, and genetic laxity of soft tissues. If the defect extends more than approximately 1 cm in chronic and/or neglected ruptures, a tendon transfer should be considered.

H. Thermann (✉) • C. Becher
International Center of Hip-, Knee- and Foot Surgery,
ATOS Clinic Heidelberg, Heidelberg, Germany
e-mail: thermann@atos.de; becher.chris@web.de

© ESSKA 2017
H. Thermann et al. (eds.), *The Achilles Tendon*, DOI 10.1007/978-3-662-54074-9_22

22.2   Operative Setup

The setup for chronic ruptures is identical to that for the endoscopic treatment of midportion Achilles tendinopathy and semi-T transfer (see Chaps. 8 and 17).

If considerable adhesions are present, especially in cases with prior operative treatment, 3.2 mm punches and a normal, stable scissor should be available in order to release the scar tissue.

A no. 11 scalpel blade is needed for the incisions of the tendon.

Special care must be taken not to get into area of the sural nerve, the peripheral lateral arterial vascularization, and the anterior neurovascular bundle.

We recommend after tendon reconstruction to apply fibrin glue (e.g., Tissucol 5 ml) and if there is the possibility for application, a PRP product, a centrifuge, and appropriate syringe to be available.

22.3   Surgical Technique

The amount of shortening should usually not exceed 1 cm (Fig. 22.1). The incisions are created proximal and distal at the ends of the defect area on the medial side and at the distal end of the lateral side (Fig. 22.2). The subcutaneous soft tissue is spread with a mosquito clamp along the dorsal portion of the tendon to create a space for endoscopy from the two medial incisions. In some cases, the use of a stable scissor is necessary for the release of scar tissue. The release is carried out from both the proximal and the distal incision. The arthroscope is inserted through the proximal incision, a 3.8 mm shaver from the distal incision. By triangulation, the shaver is brought directly into the surgical field (see Chap. 8).

A further release is performed with the shaver to ensure a free mobilization of the gastroc-soleus complex. Care must be taken not to lacerate the side branch of the fibular nerve as well as the nearby lying sural nerve on the lateral side as well as the tibial artery with its branches and the tibial nerve on the medial side, respectively.

With the no. 11 scalpel, the tendon is incised from the proximal medial and distal lateral approaches with resection of approximately 5 mm of tendon tissue each after applying the central midline cut of the tendon (Fig. 22.1). For the midline cut of the tendon, the skin incisions must be enlarged as necessary and moved as a window.

The tendon ends are fixed with non-resorbable suture material (FiberWire®, Arthrex GmbH, München) by starting with the proximal and distal central ends of the midline cut. The sutures are completed medially and laterally (Fig. 22.2). As for the central midline cut, the skin incisions must be moved as a window to have a good approach.

A framewise suture using a FiberTape (FiberTape®, Arthrex GmbH, München) to secure the sutured tendon ends is performed (Fig. 22.2) with positioning the foot in equinus position.

We recommend applying fibrin glue for sealing of the entire reconstructed area under visual control. Finally, a PRP product is injected. Optionally, an 8 mm drain can be introduced and the incisions closed in common fashion.

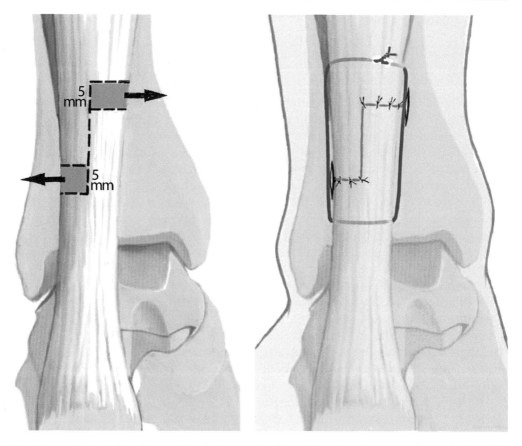

Fig. 22.1 Schematic illustration of the Achilles tendon z shortening with resection of 5 mm tendon each on the medial and lateral side

Fig. 22.2 Illustration of the sutures for re-adaption of the tendon ends, and framewise protection of the reconstructed tendon with a FiberTape®

22.4 Postoperative Care

After application of the wound dressing with cotton wool fixed with an elastic bandage, a prefabricated cardboard splint is applied in equinus position. Moderate movement exercises from 5° to 10° plantar flexion can start from the third/fourth day as tolerated by pain and swelling.

Thereafter, mild exercises in the form of a "moderate motion" are performed in plantar flexion, thus preventing the scarring of the tendon and allowing early gliding of the tendon. Lymphatic drainage and physiotherapy with motion exercises of the ankle, especially stretching the flexor chain in plantar flexion, are added.

With good wound and swelling conditions, full weight bearing is allowed in the boot (Vario-Stabil, Orthotech GmbH, 82131 Gauting-Stockdorf, Germany). After 8 weeks and ultrasound control, the patient can proceed with the physical therapy and the muscle strengthening (only in plantar flexion) in case of good graft regeneration.

Otherwise the postoperative care is comparable to that after percutaneous suturing (Chap. 2).

22.5 Pearls and Pitfalls

- A thorough mobilization of the gastroc-soleus complex is necessary to regain gliding soft tissues.
- The central proximal and distal sutures should be performed first for a good re-adaption of the tendon ends.
- In larger defect situations, a tendon transfer might be necessary.
- Patients must be informed that the longer the situation was present, the less the chances for a good recovery of muscle function.

References

1. Cannon LB, Hackney RG. Operative shortening of the elongated defunctioned tendoachillies following previous rupture. J R Nav Med Serv. 2003;89(3):139–41.
2. Maffulli N, Spiezia F, Longo UG, Denaro V. Z-shortening of healed, elongated Achilles tendon rupture. Int Orthop. 2012;36(10):2087–93.
3. Khan RJ, Fick D, Keogh A, Crawford J, Brammar T, Parker M. Treatment of acute achilles tendon ruptures. A meta-analysis of randomized, controlled trials. J Bone Joint Surg Am. 2005;87(10):2202–10.

Part VII

Biologics in Tendon Healing

Biologics in Tendon Healing: PRP/Fibrin/Stem Cells

23

Paul W. Ackermann

23.1 Introduction

Optimization of tendon healing is a complex process, which requires a perfect understanding of the sequences of the repair process and the close interaction between blood-derived cells (e.g., platelets, leukocytes, monocytes, and lymphocytes) and tissue-derived cells (e.g., macrophages, fibroblasts, myofibroblasts, endothelial cells, mast cells, and stem cells). The direct aim of the healing process is to achieve tissue integrity, homeostasis, and load-bearing capability.

The repair process can be subdivided into five important overlapping sequences: (1) induction, (2) production, (3) orchestration, (4) conduction, and (5) modification (Fig. 23.1). Biological enhancement of the healing process with novel procedures can be performed by interaction in different stages of the healing process [1].

P.W. Ackermann
Karolinska Institutet, Department of Molecular Medicine and Surgery, SE-17176 Stockholm, Sweden

Department of Orthopaedics and Sports Medicine,
Karolinska University Hospital,
SE-17176 Stockholm, Sweden
e-mail: paul.ackermann@karolinska.se

H. Thermann et al. (eds.), *The Achilles Tendon*, DOI 10.1007/978-3-662-54074-9_23

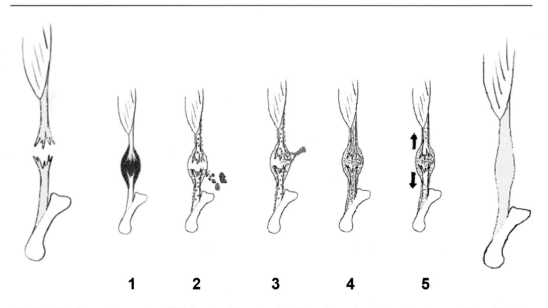

Fig. 23.1 Tendon repair overview. (1) Induction, (2) production, (3) orchestration, (4) conduction, and (5) modification of the healing process (Reproduced with permission from Ackermann [1])

23.2 Induction of the Healing Process

After tendon injury, the wound site is infiltrated with blood-derived cells, which contribute to ending of the bleeding process, clean up tissue debris, and direct further traffic by release of inflammatory mediators, e.g., cytokines, nitric oxide, and growth factors (GF). This is the initiation of the inflammatory healing phase.

23.2.1 Platelets

One of the most important blood-derived cells is platelets, which release a wide variety of growth factors at the site of tendon injury. Many of these growth factors have been demonstrated to promote repair in various soft tissue models. Thus, blood-derived cells, e.g., platelets, and the subsequently released growth factors are essential for the initiation of the healing process [2].

23.2.1.1 Can Platelet-Rich Plasma (PRP) Speed Up Tendon Healing?

Platelet-rich plasma (PRP) is derived from centrifugation of whole blood; it is the cellular component of plasma that settles after centrifugation. PRP contains numerous growth factors such as platelet-derived growth factor, vascular endothelial growth factor, insulin-like growth factor (IGF)-1, and fibroblast growth factor, which each individually has demonstrated important regulatory effects on tendon repair. Thus, PRP is believed to be able to enhance tendon healing.

In deficient healing conditions without bleeding, such as Achilles tendon disorders, e.g., tendinopathy, platelet-rich plasma (PRP) injections have become a very popular treatment alternative [3]. Thus, experimental studies have found positive effects in tendinopathy and tendon healing, possibly by PRP influencing neovascularization, collagen production, and fibroblast proliferation in the early phase of tendon healing [4–6]. However, at present the most effective dose of different growth factors in various PRP preparations and optimal treatment intervals for

enhancement of tendon repair are not even known for experimental tendon injuries.

Although many in vitro and in vivo studies suggest potentially beneficial effects of using PRP in Achilles tendon pathology, there are only a few well-conducted randomized controlled clinical trials, which show a very limited evidence of clinical advantage. Thus, at present, there are unknown variables, e.g., delivery system, local environment, receptor activation, and tendon loading, which have to be mastered before growth factor delivery therapies, e.g., PRP, can become clinically effective.

Platelet-rich plasma injection for treating tendon problems, such as tendinopathy, is a relatively new treatment method, and current evidence recommends against its clinical use and instead suggests the use of PRP in clinical studies. There is a lack of clinical RCT studies, and the majority of the studies show little or no evidence for PRP injections as treatment for tendinopathy [6]. A prospective study by De Vos et al. showed in patients with Achilles tendinopathy no more effectiveness with PRP injections compared with saline injections (placebo), while both groups also underwent an eccentric exercise program [6].

Recently, a publication in Lancet by Alsousou et al. examined tendon tissue biopsy samples from 20 patients with ruptured Achilles tendon by means of ultrasound-guided needle biopsies from the healing area of the Achilles tendon 6 weeks after treatment with PRP or placebo controls [7]. The study by Alsousou et al. demonstrated immunohistologically that locally applied PRP enhanced the maturity of the healing tendon tissues by promoting better collagen I deposition, decreased cellularity, less vascularity, and higher glycosaminoglycan content when compared with control samples. However, further work is required to determine the long-term clinical effects of the use of PRP injections.

23.2.1.2 Platelet-Rich Fibrin (PRF)

Platelet-rich fibrin (PRF) and leukocyte- and platelet-rich fibrin (L-PRF) are matrices, which consist of bioactive components of whole blood that include platelet activation and fibrin polymerization [8]. The L-PRF matrix is produced by a standard centrifugation procedure in less than 20 min. As opposed to PRP, L-PRF does not dissolve so quickly during the first hours after application [9]. Moreover, due to the primary fibrin polymerization, the stable matrix encapsulates growth factors, which allows a continuous slow release of growth factors for up to 28 days [9]. The leukocytes additionally produce a significant amount of growth factors that are known to promote healing [10].

One experimental study on Achilles tendon healing suggested that rats treated with PRF compared to those treated with PRP showed a better cellular organization when compared at 28 days after treatment [11]. Fibrin glue has been known since the 1980s for augmenting repair of the human Achilles tendon. Some authors have suggested that the use of fibrin glue could be an alternative to the traditional suture repair of ruptured Achilles tendon. However, still there are not sufficient scientific evidences to support clinical use of PRF or fibrin glue to enhance Achilles tendon healing as compared standard procedures [12].

23.3   Stimulation of Callus Production

Tissue-derived cells are attracted and transformed into myofibroblasts at the healing site by inflammatory mediators released from the blood clot. The myofibroblasts subsequently activate production of tendon callus [13]. In that way, granulation tissue, i.e., extracellular matrix and collagen type III, is formed from the tissue-derived cells that normally reside in the extrinsic peritendinous tissues and the intrinsic tissue of the epitenon and endotenon. During the first week, collagen synthesis commences and reaches its maximum by week four – the reparative, collagen-forming phase. The glycoprotein, fibronectin, acts as a chemotactic agent for fibroblasts, which are the predominant cell type for production of type III collagen. The fibroblasts respond to mechanical loading by increased production of collagen.

The tissue- and blood-derived cells that infiltrate the wound area moreover release a cascade of mediators (growth factors, cytokines, bone morphogenetic proteins (BMPs), and neuropeptides). Supplements of these factors have in numerous experimental studies demonstrated promising results for optimization of the repair process. Growth factors (GF) typically have a very short half-life in the tissues, therefore the development of a number of different methods of prolonged GF release such as GF-saturated sponges, scaffolds, and lately GF-coated sutures.

23.3.1   Insulin-Like Growth Factor (IGF)

IGF promotes cell proliferation and collagen synthesis and decreases swelling in healing tendons [14]. Experimental studies have shown higher Achilles tendon function scores and accelerated recovery in rats after IGF administration [15, 16].

23.3.2   Transforming Growth Factor-β (TGF-β)

TGF-β is profuse in healing and scar formation. Its fetal isoforms (TGF-β2 and 3) promote healing without scar tissue formation. This might be suggesting that inhibition of TGF-β1 and exogenous administration of β2 and 3 would promote healing in the absence of excessive scar tissue formation. Experimental studies have shown that TGF-β1 administration and suppression of β2 and 3 results in increased cross-sectional area but lower failure load, i.e., mechanically inferior tissue quality [17].

23.3.3   Bone Morphogenetic Proteins (BMPs)

BMPs were discovered by their ability to induce formation of bone and cartilage. In Achilles tendon healing, a local injection of each of BMP-12, BMP-13, or BMP-14 into the hematoma 6 hours after Achilles tendon transection leads to approximately 30% increase in total strength after

1 week in the rat [18]. In the rabbit, similar effects have been observed at 2 weeks [19]. BMP-12 has also been demonstrated to induce tenogenic differentiation of adipose-derived stromal cells [20].

23.3.4 Neuropeptides

In addition to growth factors, specific neuromediators, so-called neuropeptides that are released by ingrowing nerve fibers during tendon repair, have essential effects on the healing process (Fig. 23.3) [21–24]. Nerve sprouting and growth within the tendon proper is followed by a time-dependent expression of neuropeptides during the tendon healing process [24]. During inflammatory and early proliferative healing, mainly sensory neuropeptides (e.g., substance P) are released (Fig. 23.4) [24]. Subsequently, after the healing process is finished, sprouting nerve fibers within the tendon proper retract to the surrounding structures, i.e., the paratenon and surrounding loose connective tissue. Presumably, nerve retraction is also essential for healing progression.

Injections of substance P in physiological concentrations to the healing Achilles tendon have proved to enhance fibroblast aggregation, collagen production, and organization and to increase tensile strength more than 100% compared with controls [25–27]. Moreover, supplement with substance P enhanced nerve retraction.

23.3.5 Stem Cells

Since optimal delivery of growth factors as yet has been of limited clinical success, molecular approaches have been developed. Mesenchymal stem cells (MSC) [28], bone marrow stem cells (BMSC) [29], and genetically modified cells that synthesize and deliver the desired growth factor in a temporally and spatially orchestrated manner to the wound site would be a powerful means to overcome the limitations of various delivery systems [30].

Since tendon healing and tendinopathy often involves a component of failed healing, the rationale of supplementing the healing process with stem cells is an interesting and lucrative approach. Some experimental studies have shown beneficial effects on the repair process with stem cell injections; however, much regarding the type of therapy still needs to be further investigated.

Five clinical trials have reported the use of stem cells for the promotion of tendon repair (chronic tendinopathy, three; rotator cuff tear, two) with initially promising results. There are two clinical studies reporting the safety of using allogeneic stem cells for the promotion of tendon repair. Injection of allogeneic stem cells for the treatment of chronic lateral epicondylosis was reported to be safe and effectively improved elbow pain, performance, and structural defects after 1 year in a small, uncontrolled trial of 12 patients [31]. Ultrasound-guided injection of allogeneic human placenta-derived mesenchymal stromal cells was also reported to be safe in six patients with refractory Achilles tendinopathy at 4 weeks after administration. However, still the sample sizes in the clinical studies are small and mostly there were no control groups.

23.4 Orchestration of Callus Formation

During initiation of matrix production, the healing tendon proper, which normally is practically devoid of nerves and vessels (Fig. 23.2), is successively infiltrated by new nerves and vessels providing a "highway" for the delivery of essential neurovascular mediators that orchestrate and enhance the repair process (Fig. 23.3) [13, 21, 23, 24].

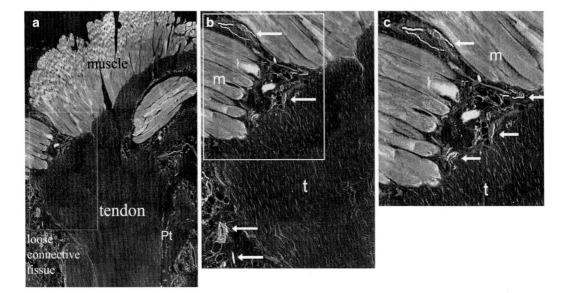

Fig. 23.2 (**a–c**). Healthy tendon neurovascular anatomy. Tendon proper (intrafascicular matrix) practically devoid of nerves and blood vessels. Overview micrographs of longitudinal sections through the Achilles tendon. Incubation with antisera to the general nerve marker PGP 9.5. Micrographs depict the proximal half of the Achilles tendon at increasing magnification in figures (**a–c**). *Arrows* denote varicosities and nerve terminals. The typical vascular localization of autonomic neuropeptides is depicted in the *lower left* (**b**), whereas the free nerve endings are a typical localization of sensory neuropeptides (**c**). The immunoreactivity is seen in the paratenon (interfascicular matrix) and surrounding loose connective tissue, whereas the proper tendinous tissue, notably, is almost devoid of nerve fibers (*pt* = paratenon) (Reproduced with permission from Ackermann et al. [23])

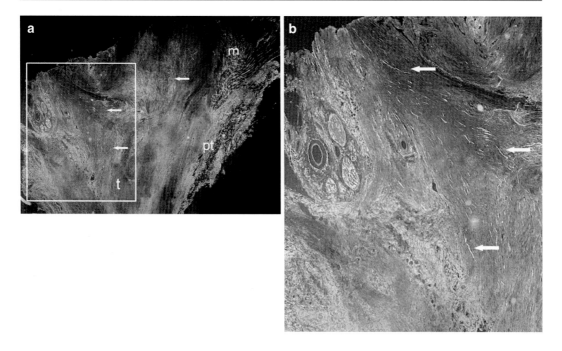

Fig. 23.3 (**a**, **b**) Tendon healing anatomy. Overview micrographs of longitudinal sections through the Achilles tendon at 2 weeks post-injury (rupture). Incubation with antisera to a nerve growth marker, GAP-43. Micrographs depict the proximal half of the Achilles tendon at increasing magnification in figures (**a**, **b**). *Arrows* denote varicosities and nerve terminals. The GAP-positive fibers, indicating wound reinnervation, are abundantly observed in the healing tendon tissue (Reproduced with permission from Ackermann et al. [23])

23.4.1 Neoinnervation and Neovascularization

New nerve ingrowth within the tendon proper, which normally is aneuronal, is followed by a time-dependent expression of neuropeptides during the tendon healing process (Fig. 23.4) [21, 23, 24]. During the inflammatory and early proliferative phase, i.e., 2–6 weeks after injury, there is a striking increased occurrence of sensory neuropeptides, substance P (SP), and calcitonin gene-related peptide (CGRP) in the healing tendon tissue. Thus, SP is known to enhance angiogenesis [32] and improves repair by homing stromal stem cells to the site of injury [33].

However, for healing to progress, the ingrown nerves and vessels have to retract, a process which is promoted by adequate mechanical stimuli. In case of tendinopathy, an increased number of vessels and sensory nerves with elevated SP levels have been observed within the proper tendon, indicating an unaccomplished healing process. Thus, signals that regulate nerve and blood vessel retraction are critical in the understanding of tendinopathy prevention. Factors that may regulate nerve retraction and are released at mechanical stimulus during tendon healing include IL-6 family members [34–36], neurotrophic factors [37], glutamate [38], and their receptors [39–42].

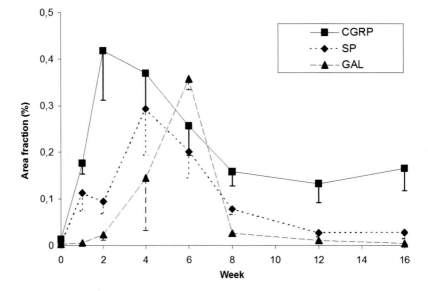

Fig. 23.4 Tendon healing – neuropeptide expression. Area within tendon proper occupied by nerve fibers (%) immunoreactive to neuropeptides SP, CGRP, and GAL in relation to the total healing area, over 16 weeks post-tendon injury (mean ± SEM) (Reproduced with permission from [24])

23.5 Conduction of Cell and Tissue Ingrowth

A prerequisite for healing to commence is an existing and functioning tissue matrix into which cells, vessels, and nerves can grow in and where production of new granulation tissue can occur. If a tissue defect exists, the repair process will be prolonged or will not be able to take place at all. Hence, in conservative as well as in surgical treatment of patients with tendon injuries, it is an important principle to bring the disrupted tendon parts close together for regulation of fibril fusion and new tissue ingrowth. Small-sized defects can mostly be managed by autologous methods, i.e., repair by remaining tendon tissue, flap techniques, or tendon grafts. Larger defects do sometimes need free tendon grafts (e.g., semitendinosus tendon) and/or scaffolding techniques – either biogenic or synthetic (e.g., bioresorbable polymers) scaffolds. At present, autologous graft is still the gold standard, while the development of new biogenic or synthetic scaffolds is still under investigation [14].

23.6 Modification of the Healing Callus

23.6.1 Mobilization

Mobilization leading to mechanical tendon loading is the most well-known extrinsic factor adapted to regulate tendon protein synthesis and degradation [43]. One exercise bout in human tendons activates an initial increase in both the synthesis and degradation of collagen. The initial loss of collagen after loading is thus over time ensued by a net gain in collagen.

During the healing process, the mechanical loading is even more important for tendon tissue properties. Increasing mechanical loading activates myofibroblasts and fibroblasts to increase the production of collagen type I to increase the callus size and enhance the capacity to withstand high mechanical load. With loading of the tendon, the orientation of fibroblasts and collagen changes to the longitudinal axis of the tendon by 4 weeks after injury. By 4 weeks, the mechanical strength of the repairing tendon increases, as there is consolidation and remodeling of the maturing granulation tissue under tension, and the collagen synthesis under load changes from type III to type I. Various factors influence the rate and quality of tendon healing. The most important is the mechanical tension across the repair which speeds realignment of collagen fibers, increases tensile strength, and minimizes deformation at the repair site [44]. Early mobilization accelerates the nerve plasticity, i.e., nerve regeneration, expression of neuromediators and their receptors, and nerve retraction (Figs. 23.2 and 23.3) [41, 45].

23.6.2 Immobilization

Mechanical stimuli promote tendon repair, while immobilization is detrimental for healing (Fig. 23.5). In a rat model with plaster cast immobilization of the hind limb after Achilles tendon rupture, the ultimate tensile strength was reduced 80% at 2 weeks post-rupture compared with a freely mobilized group [46]. Moreover, in the same model of hind limb immobilized rats, mRNA expression of essential sensory neuropeptide receptors (NK-1, RAMP), growth factors (BDNF, bFGF), and extracellular matrix molecules (collagen type I and III, versican, decorin, biglycan) were all downregulated at 2 weeks post-rupture [37, 41]. In the same studies, it was demonstrated that a shorter period of immobilization, i.e., 1 week, did not affect mRNA expression of the abovementioned molecules. These reports support the notion that prolonged immobilization post-injury hampers the healing process by compromising the up-regulation of repair gene expression in the healing tendon. Moreover, the data also suggest that endogenous, as well as exogenously given, growth factors PRP-therapies may not be effective until mechanical stimulation is initiated, since their receptors are not up-regulated [37].

23.6.3 Mechanical Stimulation During Immobilization

One novel method of applying mechanical stimulation to an immobilized tendon could be applied by using adjuvant intermittent pneumatic compression (IPC). IPC, which clinically is adapted to prevent thrombosis and increase blood circulation [47], has experimentally proven positive effects on wound and fracture healing [46, 48], although the mechanisms are still largely unknown. Recently, however, IPC was demonstrated to enhance neurovascular ingrowth in a tendon repair model such as to increase the expression of sensory neuropeptides by up to 100% [49]. In the same model, IPC was able during immobilization to improve maximum force by 65%, energy 168%, organized collagen diameter 50%, and collagen III occurrence 150% compared with immobilization only [46] (Fig. 23.5). Whether IPC can reverse the negative effects of immobilization in patients still needs to be further explored.

Group	Intact[a]	Mobilization	Immobilization		Immobilization + IPC treatment	
Parameter	Mean ± SEM	Mean ± SEM	Mean ± SEM	p-Level[c]	Mean ± SEM	p-Level[c]
Max force (N)	43.0 ± 4.2	46.9 ± 3	9.5 ± 1.4	<0.001	15.7 ± 2.4	<0.001
Energy (J)	82.9 ± 4.2	99 ± 13.5	25 ± 9.7	0.005	67 ± 12.5	0.109
Stiffness (N/mm)	13.1 ± 1.2	16.6 ± 1	3.8 ± 0.4	<0.001	5 ± 0.6	<0.001
Length (mm)	8.9 ± 0.4	14.7 ± 0.9	11.4 ± 1	0.025	14.3 ± 0.5	0.567
Cross area (mm^2)	3.0 ± 0.5	16.2 ± 1.9	8.6 ± 0.5	0.013	11.3 ± 1.6	0.050
Stress (N/mm^2)	17.5 ± 3.9	3.3 ± 0.3	1.1 ± 0.2	0.002	1.5 ± 0.2	0.001
Organized collagen (%)	100	53 ± 3.1	27 ± 3.5	0.004	40 ± 2.5	0.017
Collagen III-LI (%)	NA[b]	5.9 ± 1.9	1.0 ± 0.1	0.004	2.5 ± 0.5	0.052

Fig. 23.5 Biomechanical healing properties during mobilization/immobilization. At 2 weeks post-tendon rupture, maximum force at failure of freely mobilized rats already reached the values of "normal" uninjured. Compared to mobilization, 2 weeks of immobilization caused significantly lower values ($p \leq 0.05$) for all parameters. IPC treatment, however, seems to counteract the effects of immobilization (Reproduced with permission from Schizas et al. [46])

Conclusion

Several novel and modified versions of old therapies rapidly become available for the use of enhancing tendon repair. Although novel tissue engineering and tissue regenerative techniques addressing tendon repair seem promising, these are not yet ready for routine clinical use. Such methods include molecular approaches by which PRP, PRF, and fibrin glue, including stem cells, synthesize growth factors, or other mediators needed for progression of failed healing.

Having this said, I also want to clearly state that – the future lies in biological augmentation of tendon healing – once the correct indications are there, the correct formulations are understood, and the adjuvant treatments during the different healing phases are correctly applied.

References

1. Ackermann PW. Healing and repair mechanisms. London: DJO Publications; 2014.
2. Broughton 2nd G, Janis JE, Attinger CE. Wound healing: an overview. Plast Reconstr Surg. 2006; 117(7 Suppl):1e-S–32e-S.
3. Andia I, Sanchez M, Maffulli N. Tendon healing and platelet-rich plasma therapies. Expert Opin Biol Ther. 10(10):1415–26.
4. Kaux JF, Drion PV, Colige A, et al. Effects of platelet-rich plasma (PRP) on the healing of Achilles tendons of rats. Wound Repair Regen. 2012;20(5):748–56.
5. Lyras DN, Kazakos K, Verettas D, et al. The influence of platelet-rich plasma on angiogenesis during the early phase of tendon healing. Foot Ankle Int. 2009;30(11):1101–6.
6. Paoloni J, De Vos RJ, Hamilton B, et al. Platelet-rich plasma treatment for ligament and tendon injuries. Clin J Sport Med. 2011;21(1):37–45.
7. Alsousou J, Thompson M, Harrison P, et al. Effect of platelet-rich plasma on healing tissues in acute ruptured Achilles tendon: a human immunohistochemistry study. Lancet. 2015;385 Suppl 1:S19.
8. Dohan DM, Choukroun J, Diss A, et al. Platelet-rich fibrin (PRF): a second-generation platelet concentrate. Part I: technological concepts and evolution. Oral Surg Oral Med Oral Pathol Oral Radiol Endod. 2006;101(3):e37–44.
9. Zumstein MA, Berger S, Schober M, et al. Leukocyte- and platelet-rich fibrin (L-PRF) for long-term delivery of growth factor in rotator cuff repair: review, preliminary results and future directions. Curr Pharm Biotechnol. 2012;13(7):1196–206.
10. Dohan Ehrenfest DM, de Peppo GM, Doglioli P, et al. Slow release of growth factors and thrombospondin-1 in Choukroun's platelet-rich fibrin (PRF): a gold standard to achieve for all surgical platelet concentrates technologies. Growth Factors. 2009;27(1):63–9.
11. Dietrich F, Duré G L, P Klein C, et al. Platelet-rich fibrin promotes an accelerated healing of Achilles tendon when compared to platelet-rich plasma in rat. World J Plast Surg. 2015;4(2):101–9.
12. Knobe M, Gradl G, Klos K, et al. Is percutaneous suturing superior to open fibrin gluing in acute Achilles tendon rupture? Int Orthop. 2015;39(3):535–42.
13. Martin P. Wound healing–aiming for perfect skin regeneration. Science (New York). 1997;276(5309): 75–81.
14. Longo UG, Lamberti A, Maffulli N, et al. Tissue engineered biological augmentation for tendon healing: a systematic review. Br Med Bull. 2011;98:31–59.
15. Tang Y, Leng Q, Xiang X, et al. Use of ultrasound-targeted microbubble destruction to transfect IGF-1 cDNA to enhance the regeneration of rat wounded Achilles tendon in vivo. Gene Ther. 2015;22(8):610–8.
16. Kurtz CA, Loebig TG, Anderson DD, et al. Insulin-like growth factor I accelerates functional recovery from Achilles tendon injury in a rat model. Am J Sports Med. 1999;27(3):363–9.
17. Molloy T, Wang Y, Murrell G. The roles of growth factors in tendon and ligament healing. Sports Med. 2003;33(5):381–94.
18. Forslund C, Rueger D, Aspenberg P. A comparative dose-response study of cartilage-derived morphogenetic protein (CDMP)-1, -2 and -3 for tendon healing in rats. J Orthop Res. 2003;21(4):617–21.
19. Forslund C, Aspenberg P. Improved healing of transected rabbit Achilles tendon after a single injection of cartilage-derived morphogenetic protein-2. Am J Sports Med. 2003;31(4):555–9.
20. Shen H, Gelberman RH, Silva MJ, et al. BMP12 induces tenogenic differentiation of adipose-derived stromal cells. PLoS One. 2013;8(10):e77613.
21. Ackermann PW, Franklin SL, Dean BJ, et al. Neuronal pathways in tendon healing and tendinopathy–update. Front Biosci. 2014;19:1251–78.
22. Ackermann PW. Neuronal regulation of tendon homoeostasis. Int J Exp Pathol. 2013;94:271–86.
23. Ackermann PW, Ahmed M, Kreicbergs A. Early nerve regeneration after achilles tendon rupture–a prerequisite for healing? A study in the rat. J Orthop Res. 2002;20(4):849–56.
24. Ackermann PW, Li J, Lundeberg T, et al. Neuronal plasticity in relation to nociception and healing of rat achilles tendon. J Orthop Res. 2003;21(3):432–41.
25. Burssens P, Steyaert A, Forsyth R, et al. Exogenously administered substance P and neutral endopeptidase inhibitors stimulate fibroblast proliferation, angiogenesis

and collagen organization during Achilles tendon healing. Foot Ankle Int. 2005;26(10):832–9.

26. Carlsson O, Schizas N, Li J, et al. Substance P injections enhance tissue proliferation and regulate sensory nerve ingrowth in rat tendon repair. Scand J Med Sci Sports. 2011;21(4):562–9.

27. Steyaert AE, Burssens PJ, Vercruysse CW, et al. The effects of substance P on the biomechanic properties of ruptured rat Achilles' tendon. Arch Phys Med Rehabil. 2006;87(2):254–8.

28. Nourissat G, Diop A, Maurel N, et al. Mesenchymal stem cell therapy regenerates the native bone-tendon junction after surgical repair in a degenerative rat model. PLoS One. 2010;5(8):e12248.

29. Okamoto N, Kushida T, Oe K, et al. Treating Achilles tendon rupture in rats with bone-marrow-cell transplantation therapy. J Bone Joint Surg Am. 2010;92(17): 2776–84.

30. Ackermann PW, Salo PT, Hart DA. Gene therapy. In: Van Dijk N, Karlsson J, Maffulli N, editors. Achilles tendinopathy current concept. London: DJO Publications; 2010. p. 165–75.

31. Lee SY, Kim W, Lim C, et al. Treatment of lateral epicondylosis by using allogeneic adipose-derived mesenchymal stem cells: a Pilot Study. Stem Cells. 2015;33(10):2995–3005.

32. Haegerstrand A, Dalsgaard CJ, Jonzon B, et al. Calcitonin gene-related peptide stimulates proliferation of human endothelial cells. Proc Natl Acad Sci U S A. 1990;87(9):3299–303.

33. Hong HS, Lee J, Lee E, et al. A new role of substance P as an injury-inducible messenger for mobilization of CD29(+) stromal-like cells. Nat Med. 2009;15(4): 425–35.

34. Legerlotz K, Jones ER, Screen HR, et al. Increased expression of IL-6 family members in tendon pathology. Rheumatology. 2012;51(7):1161–5.

35. Ackermann PW, Domeij-Arverud E, Leclerc P, et al. Anti-inflammatory cytokine profile in early human tendon repair. Knee Surg Sports Traumatol Arthrosc. 2013;21(8):1801–6.

36. Andersen MB, Pingel J, Kjaer M, et al. Interleukin-6: a growth factor stimulating collagen synthesis in human tendon. J Appl Physiol. 2011;110(6):1549–54.

37. Bring D, Reno C, Renstrom P, et al. Prolonged immobilization compromises up-regulation of repair genes after tendon rupture in a rat model. Scand J Med Sci Sports. 2010;20(3):411–7.

38. Greve K, Domeij-Arverud E, Labruto F, et al. Metabolic activity in early tendon repair can be enhanced by intermittent pneumatic compression. Scand J Med Sci Sports. 2012;22(4):e55–63.

39. Schizas N, Lian O, Frihagen F, et al. Coexistence of up-regulated NMDA receptor 1 and glutamate on nerves, vessels and transformed tenocytes in tendinopathy. Scand J Med Sci Sports. 2010;20(2): 208–15.

40. Schizas N, Weiss R, Lian O, et al. Glutamate receptors in tendinopathic patients. J Orthop Res. 2012; 30(9):1447–52.

41. Bring DKI, Reno C, Renstrom P, et al. Joint immobilization reduces the expression of sensory neuropeptide receptors and impairs healing after tendon rupture in a rat model. J Orthop Res. 2009;27(2):274–80.

42. Hou ST, Jiang SX, Smith RA. Permissive and repulsive cues and signalling pathways of axonal outgrowth and regeneration. Int Rev Cell Mol Biol. 2008; 267:125–81.

43. Magnusson SP, Langberg H, Kjaer M. The pathogenesis of tendinopathy: balancing the response to loading. Nat Rev Rheumatol. 2010;6(5):262–8.

44. Gelberman RH, Manske PR, Akeson WH, et al. Flexor tendon repair. J Orthop Res. 1986;4(1):119–28.

45. Bring DKI, Kreicbergs A, Renstrom PAFH, et al. Physical activity modulates nerve plasticity and stimulates repair after Achilles tendon rupture. J Orthop Res. 2007;25(2):164–72.

46. Schizas N, Li J, Andersson T, et al. Compression therapy promotes proliferative repair during rat Achilles tendon immobilization. J Orthop Res. 2010;28(7):852–8.

47. Kakkos SK, Caprini JA, Geroulakos G, et al. Combined intermittent pneumatic leg compression and pharmacological prophylaxis for prevention of venous thromboembolism in high-risk patients. Cochrane Database Syst Rev. 2008;4:CD005258.

48. Khanna A, Gougoulias N, Maffulli N. Intermittent pneumatic compression in fracture and soft-tissue injuries healing. Br Med Bull. 2008;88(1):147–56.

49. Dahl J, Li J, Bring DK, et al. Intermittent pneumatic compression enhances neurovascular ingrowth and tissue proliferation during connective tissue healing: a study in the rat. J Orthop Res. 2007;25(9):1185–92.

Index

A

Achilles tendon lengthening
    gastrocnemius slide, 119–122
    minimally invasive lengthening, 113–118
Achilles tendon rupture
    endoscopic-assisted free graft technique with semi-T
        transfer, 99–102
    endoscopic flexor hallucis longus tendon transfer,
        103–109
    free/turndown gastrocnemius flap augmentation, 81–83
    ipsilateral free semitendinosus tendon graft with
        interference screw fixation, 93–97
    minimally invasive peroneus brevis tendon transfer,
        89–92
    open reconstruction with gastrocnemius V-Y
        advancement, 75–80
Achilles tendon shortening
    endoscopically assisted mini-open technique, 129–132
    healed achilles tendon rupture, Z shortening of, 125–128
Achillon®, 30
    indication and diagnosis, 27
    operative setup, 28
    postoperative care, 30
    surgical technique, 28–30
Achillon device, 28, 29
Acute Achilles tendon ruptures
    Achillon®, 27–30
    distal Achilles tendon rupture repair, 31–36
    lace technique, 21–24
    open standard technique, 3–5
    percutaneous suturing with double-knot technique,
        7–13
    three-bundle technique, 15–19
Allis clamp, 77. *See* Kocher clamp
Ankle-foot orthosis (AFO) bracing, 75
Antibiotic prophylaxis, 22, 70
Arthrex®, 31
Arthroscopy, 46, 47, 104
Aspirin, 72

B

Beath pin, 90, 95, 105
Bone morphogenetic proteins (BMPs), 138–139
Bunnell sutures, 17

C

Calcified insertional Achilles tendinopathy, open
        technique for, 72
    indication and diagnosis, 69
    operative setup, 69–70
    postoperative care, 72
Calf squeeze testing, 27
Callus formation, orchestration, 140–142
Callus production
    BMPs, 138–139
    IGF, 138
    neuropeptides, 139
    stem cells, 139
    TGF-β, 138
    tissue-derived cells, 138
Controlled ankle motion (CAM) boot, 75, 80

D

Delayed Achilles tendon rupture
    endoscopic-assisted free graft technique, 99–102
    endoscopic flexor hallucis longus tendon transfer,
        103–109
    free hamstring open augmentation, 85–88
    free/turndown gastrocnemius flap augmentation, 81–83
    ipsilateral free semitendinosus tendon graft, 93–97
    minimally invasive peroneus brevis tendon transfer,
        89–92
Distal Achilles tendon rupture repair, 36
    indications and diagnosis, 31–32
    operative setup, 32
    postoperative care, 35
    surgical technique, 33–35
Double-knot technique, percutaneous suturing with, 13
    indication and diagnosis, 7
    operative setup, 8
    postoperative care, 12
    surgical technique
        equinus position, 8, 11
        FiberTape, 8–10
        lateral strand, pulled out, 8, 11
        medial and lateral longitudinal incisions, 8, 9
        rupture site, medial incision at, 8, 10
        tape, crosswise pulled back, 12
Dynamic clinic testing, 53

© ESSKA 2017
H. Thermann et al. (eds.), *The Achilles Tendon*, DOI 10.1007/978-3-662-54074-9

E
Ellis clamp, 100
Endoscopic debridement, 49
    chronic ruptures, degenerative areas, 99, 100
    indication and diagnosis, 45
    operative setup, 46
    postoperative care, 49
    surgical technique, 46–48
Endoscopic flexor hallucis longus (FHL) tendon transfer, 109
    indication and diagnosis, 103–104
    operative setup, 104
    postoperative care, 109
    surgical technique, 105–108
Endoscopic technique
    free graft technique, 99–102
    mini-open technique, 129–132
    noncalcified tendinopathy, 61–67
Epitendinal crisscross technique, 4
Ethibond, 94
3.0 Ethilon suture, 63, 78

F
Fascia cruris, 33, 36, 82, 116, 117
FiberTape, 8–10, 33, 34, 100, 102, 130, 131
FiberWire, 78, 100
Fibrin glue, 8, 12, 13, 46, 99, 130, 138
Flexor hallucis longus (FHL) tendon transfer,
            endoscopic, 109
    indication and diagnosis, 103–104
    operative setup, 104
    postoperative care, 109
    surgical technique, 105–108
Free hamstring open augmentation, 88
    indication and diagnosis, 85
    operative setup, 86
    postoperative care, 88
    surgical technique, 86, 87
Free/turndown gastrocnemius flap augmentation, 83
    indication and diagnosis, 81
    operative setup, 82
    post-operative care, 83
    surgical technique, 82, 83

G
Gastrocnemius contracture, 113, 118, 119
Gastrocnemius fascia, 76, 77, 79, 120
Gastrocnemius flap augmentation, free/turndown, 83
    indication and diagnosis, 81
    operative setup, 82
    post-operative care, 83
    surgical technique, 82, 83
Gastrocnemius lengthening, 118
    indication and diagnosis, 113–115
    operative setup, 116
    post-operative care, 118
    surgical technique, 116–118
Gastrocnemius slide, 122
    indication and diagnosis, 119

    operative setup, 119
    postoperative care, 122
    surgical technique, 120, 121
Gastrocnemius V-Y advancement, open reconstruction
            with, 80
    indication and diagnosis, 75–76
    operative setup, 77
    postoperative care, 80
    surgical technique, 77–79
Gracilis tendon, 86, 88

H
Haglund's deformity, 53–55, 58, 70–72
Healed Achilles tendon rupture, Z shortening of, 128
    indication and diagnosis, 125
    operative setup, 126
    postoperative care, 128
    surgical technique, 126–127
Healing callus
    immobilization, 143
    mechanical stimulation, 144
    mobilization, 143
Hindfoot instability, 53

I
Iatrogenic nerve injury, 105–107
IGF. *See* Insulin-like growth factor (IGF)
Immobilization
    CAM, 75
    healing callus, 143
    mechanical stimulation during, 144
Insertional tendinopathy
    endoscopic technique, 61–67
    open standard technique, 69–72
    open technique, 53–59
Insulin-like growth factor (IGF), 138
Intermittent pneumatic compression (IPC), 144
Ipsilateral free semitendinosus tendon graft, 94
    indication and diagnosis, 93–94
    operative setup, 94
    post-operative care, 97
    surgical technique, 94–96

K
Kager fat pad, 61
Kessler suturing technique, 4, 82, 126, 127
Knee-flexion test, 129
Knotless intra-osseous repair, SwiveLock suture,
            33, 34
Kocher clamp, 33, 77
Krackow suture technique, 31, 70, 71, 78, 100

L
Lace technique, 24
    indication and diagnosis, 21
    operative setup, 22

postoperative care, 24
surgical technique, 22–24
Leukocyte-and platelet-rich fibrin (L-PRF), 137–138
Longitudinal tenotomies, 40, 42, 45
Lymphatic drainage
   endoscopically assisted mini-open technique, 132
   endoscopic debridement, 49
   gastrocnemius slide, 122
   insertional tendinopathy, 102
   lace technique, 24
   open technique, insertional tendinopathy, 59

M
Magnetic resonance imaging (MRI)
   endoscopic-assisted free graft technique, 99, 100
   endoscopic debridement, 46
   endoscopic technique, 61
   open reconstruction with gastrocnemius V-Y
      advancement, 75
   open technique
      calcified insertional Achilles tendinopathy, 69
      insertional tendinopathy, 53, 54
   percutaneous suturing with double-knot
      technique, 12
   three-bundle technique, 15
Mason-Allen technique, 22
Mayo needle, 33, 34, 86
Mepore, 127
Mid-portion Achilles tendinopathy
   endoscopic debridement, 45–49
   open debridement, 39–43
Minimally invasive procedures
   lengthening, 113–118
   peroneus brevis tendon transfer, 89–92
Mini-open technique, endoscopically assisted, 132
   indication and diagnosis, 129
   operative setup, 130
   postoperative care, 132
   surgical technique, 130, 131
Mosquito clamp, 46, 47, 63, 100, 130
MRI. *See* Magnetic resonance imaging (MRI)

N
Neoinnervation, callus formation, 142
Neovascularization, 142
Neuropeptides, 139
Noncalcified tendinopathy, endoscopic technique, 67
   indication and diagnosis, 61, 62
   operative setup, 62
   postoperative care, 67
   surgical technique, 63–66
No-touch technique, 77, 80

O
Open debridement, mid-portion Achilles tendinopathy, 43
   indication and diagnosis, 39–40
   operative setup, 40
   post-operative care, 43

surgical technique, 40–42
Open reconstruction with gastrocnemius V-Y
   advancement, 80
   indication and diagnosis, 75–76
   operative setup, 77
   postoperative care, 80
   surgical technique, 77–79
Open standard technique
   acute Achilles tendon ruptures, 3–5
   for calcified insertional Achilles tendinopathy,
      69–72
   insertional tendinopathy, 53–59

P
PEEK suture anchor. *See* Polyethylene ether ketone
      (PEEK) suture anchor
Percutaneous Achilles Repair System (PARS),
      31, 33
Percutaneous suture, 7, 34
   with double-knot technique, 13
      indication and diagnosis, 7
      operative setup, 8
      postoperative care, 12
      surgical technique, 8–12
Peroneus brevis tendon transfer, minimally
      invasive, 92
   indication and diagnosis, 89–90
   operative setup, 90
   postoperative care, 92
   surgical technique, 90–91
Physiotherapy
   distal Achilles tendon rupture, 35
   endoscopically assisted mini-open technique, 132
   endoscopic-assisted free graft technique, 102
   endoscopic debridement, 49
   free hamstring open augmentation, 88
   gastrocnemius slide, 122
   healed Achilles tendon rupture, Z shortening, 128
   lace technique, 24
   minimally invasive lengthening, 113
   open technique, insertional tendinopathy, 59
Platelet-rich plasma (PRP) product, 12, 46, 100, 130,
      137–138
Polyethylene ether ketone (PEEK) suture anchor, 33

R
Redon drainage, 22
Retractor, 16, 17
Retrocalcaneal bursitis, 61

S
Silfverskiöld's test, 83, 113, 114
SP. *See* Substance P (SP)
Stem cells, 139
Steri-Strips, 22, 55, 91, 95, 127
Substance P (SP), 139, 142
Superficial fascia, 120
SwiveLock suture anchors, 33, 34

T
Tendinopathic tendon, 40
Tendon healing
    callus formation, orchestration of, 140–142
    callus production, stimulation of
        BMPs, 138–139
        IGF, 138
        neuropeptides, 139
        stem cells, 139
        TGF-β, 138
        tissue-derived cells, 138
    cell conduction and tissue ingrowth, 143
    healing callus, modification
        immobilization, 143
        mechanical stimulation, 144
        mobilization, 143
    induction, platelets, 137–138
    optimization, 135
    repair process, 135, 136
Tendon transfer
    endoscopic FHL, 103–109
    minimally invasive peroneus brevis, 89–92
TGF-β. *See* Transforming growth factor-β (TGF-β)
Three-bundle technique, 19
    indication and diagnosis, 15, 16
    operative setup, 16
    postoperative care, 19
    surgical technique, 17, 18
Tissue ingrowth, 143
Transforming growth factor-β (TGF-β), 138
Trans-osseous technique, 33
Transverse coronal tenotomies, 86
Turndown gastrocnemius flap augmentation, 83
    indication and diagnosis, 81
    operative setup, 82
    post-operative care, 83
    surgical technique, 82, 83
Two-portal hindfoot technique, 63, 64

U
Ultrasound, 75
    Achillon®, 27
    endoscopic technique, 61
    open reconstruction with gastrocnemius V-Y
        advancement, 75
    percutaneous suturing with double-knot technique, 12
    stem cells, 139

V
Vario-Stabil, 12

W
Whip suture, 86, 87, 105–107, 109
Wound healing, 5, 24, 55

X
X-ray
    open reconstruction with gastrocnemius V-Y
        advancement, 76
    open technique, insertional tendinopathy, 53
    three-bundle technique, 15

Z
Z shortening, healed Achilles tendon rupture, 128
    indication and diagnosis, 125
    operative setup, 126
    postoperative care, 128
    surgical technique, 126–127